Management of Complex Wounds

Guest Editor

JANET FOSTER, PhD, APRN, CNS, CCRN

CRITICAL CARE NURSING CLINICS OF NORTH AMERICA

www.ccnursing.theclinics.com

Consulting Editor
JANET FOSTER, PhD, APRN, CNS, CCRN

June 2012 • Volume 24 • Number 2

SAUNDERS an imprint of ELSEVIER, Inc.

W.B. SAUNDERS COMPANY
A Division of Elsevier Inc.

Elsevier Inc., 1600 John F. Kennedy Blvd., Suite 1800, Philadelphia, PA 19103-2899

http://www.theclinics.com

CRITICAL CARE NURSING CLINICS OF NORTH AMERICA Volume 24, Number 2
June 2012 ISSN 0899-5885, ISBN-13: 978-1-4557-4550-0

Editor: Katie Hartner
Developmental Editor: Donald E. Mumford

Critical Care Nursing Clinics of North America (ISSN 0899-5885) is published quarterly by Elsevier Inc., 360 Park Avenue South, New York, NY 10010-1710. Months of issue are March, June, September, and December. Business and Editorial Offices: 1600 John F. Kennedy Blvd., Suite 1800, Philadelphia, PA 19103-2899. Periodicals postage paid at New York, NY and additional mailing offices. Subscription prices are $144.00 per year for US individuals, $296.00 per year for US institutions, $76.00 per year for US students and residents, $192.00 per year for Canadian individuals, $371.00 per year for Canadian institutions, $219.00 per year for international individuals, $371.00 per year for international institutions and $111.00 per year for Canadian and foreign students/residents. To receive student/resident rate, orders must be accompanied by name of affiliated institution, data of term, and the *signature* of program/ residency coordinator on institution letterhead. Orders will be billed at individual rate until proof of status is received. Foreign air speed delivery is included in all *Clinics* subscription prices. All prices are subject to change without notice. **POSTMASTER:** Send address changes to *Critical Care Nursing Clinics of North America*, Elsevier Health Sciences Division, Subscription Customer Service, 3251 Riverport Lane, Maryland Heights, MO 63043. **Customer Service: 1-800-654-2452 (US and Canada); 314-447-8871 (outside US and Canada). Fax: 314-447-8029. E-mail: JournalsCustomerService-usa@elsevier.com (for print support) and JournalsOnlineSupport-usa@elsevier.com (for online support).**

Reprints. For copies of 100 or more of articles in this publication, please contact the Commercial Reprints Department, Elsevier Inc., 360 Park Avenue South, New York, New York, 10010-1710; Tel.: (212) 633-3813, Fax: (212) 462-1935, and E-mail: reprints@elsevier.com.

Critical Care Nursing Clinics of North America is covered in *MEDLINE/PubMed (Index Medicus), International Nursing Index, Nursing Citation Index, Cumulative Index to Nursing and Allied Health Literature,* and *RNdex Top 100.*

Printed and bound by CPI Group (UK) Ltd, Croydon, CR0 4YY
Transferred to Digital Print 2012

Contributors

CONSULTING EDITOR

JANET FOSTER, PhD, APRN, CNS, CCRN
Texas Woman's University, College of Nursing, Houston, Texas

GUEST EDITOR

JAN FOSTER, PhD, APRN, CNS, CCRN
President, Nursing Inquiry and Intervention, Inc., The Woodlands; Associate Professor, Texas Woman's University, College of Nursing, Houston, Texas

AUTHORS

SAMUEL B. ADAMS Jr, MD
Assistant Professor, Division of Orthopaedic Surgery; Director of Foot and Ankle Research, Duke University Medical Center, Durham, North Carolina

ADRIAN BARBUL, MD, FACS
Chairman, Department of Surgery, Sinai Hospital of Baltimore, Baltimore, Maryland; Surgeon-in-Chief, Hackensack University Medical Center, Hackensack, New York

JANICE M. BEITZ, PhD, RN, CS, CNOR, CWOCN
Associate Professor; Director of Nursing Certificate and Distributive Learning Programs; WOCNEP Co-Director, School of Nursing, La Salle University, Philadelphia, Pennsylvania

ROBERT F. DIEGELMANN, PhD
Professor of Biochemistry and Molecular Biology, Virginia Commonwealth University Medical Center, Richmond, Virginia

MARK E. EASLEY, MD
Assistant Professor, Division of Orthopaedic Surgery, Duke University Medical Center, Durham, North Carolina

JEFFREY B. FRIEDRICH, MD, FACS
Assistant Professor of Surgery and Orthopedics, University of Washington, Harborview Medical Center, Seattle, Washington

R. GLENN GASTON, MD
Chief of Hand Surgery, Carolinas Medical Centre; OrthoCarolina, Charlotte, North Carolina

STEPHANIE R. GOLDBERG, MD
Assistant Professor, Department of Surgery, Virginia Commonwealth University Medical Center, West Hospital, Richmond, Virginia

JEAN-PHILIPPE GOUIN, PhD
Assistant Professor, Department of Psychology, Concordia University, Montreal, Quebec, Canada

JANICE K. KIECOLT-GLASER, PhD
Distinguished University Professor; S. Robert Davis Chair of Medicine; Professor of Psychiatry and Psychology, Department of Psychology, The Ohio State University; Institute for Behavioral Medicine Research; Department of Psychiatry, The Ohio State University College of Medicine, Columbus, Ohio

MARSHALL A. KUREMSKY, MD
Department of Orthopedics, Carolinas Medical Center, Charlotte, North Carolina

INNEKE E. DE LAET, MD
Intensive Care Unit, ZiekenhuisNetwerk Antwerpen, Campus Stuivenberg, Antwerpen, Belgium

MANU L.N.G. MALBRAIN, MD, PhD
Past President and Treasurer, World Society on Abdominal Compartment Syndrome; Chairman, Working Group on Abdominal Problems (WGAP) within ESICM POIC section; World Society for the Abdominal Compartment Syndrome; ICU Director, Intensive Care Unit, ZiekenhuisNetwerk Antwerpen, Campus Stuivenberg, Antwerpen, Belgium

ARTHUR MANOLI II, MD
Director, Michigan International Foot and Ankle Center, Pontiac, Michigan

VINCENT J. MARKOVCHICK, MD, FAAEM
Professor Emeritus, Department of Emergency Medicine, University of Colorado School of Medicine, Denver, Colorado

MARIA E. MOREIRA, MD
Program Director, Residency in Emergency Medicine; Staff Physician, Denver Health Medical Center; Assistant Professor, Department of Emergency Medicine, University of Colorado School of Medicine, Denver, Colorado

MARK D. PERRY, MD
Associate Professor, Department of Orthopaedic Surgery, University of Texas Southwestern Medical Center, Dallas, Texas

VANI J. SABESAN, MD
Resident, Division of Orthopaedic Surgery, Duke University Medical Center, Durham, North Carolina

ALEXANDER Y. SHIN, MD
Professor, Department of Orthopedic Surgery, Mayo Clinic, Rochester, Minnesota

JEREMY Z. WILLIAMS, MD
Department of Surgery, Johns Hopkins Medical School, Sinai Hospital of Baltimore, Baltimore, Maryland

Contents

Surgeons often care for patients with conditions of abnormal wound healing, which include conditions of excessive wound healing, such as fibrosis, adhesions, and contractures, as well as conditions of inadequate wound healing, such as chronic nonhealing ulcers, recurrent hernias, and wound dehiscences. Despite many recent advances in the field, which have highlighted the importance of adjunct therapies in maximizing the healing potential, conditions of abnormal wound healing continue to cause significant cost, morbidity, and mortality. To understand how conditions of abnormal wound healing can be corrected, it is important to first understand the basic principles of wound healing.

Wound healing and its corresponding relationship to nutrition has been acknowledged for centuries. Only more recently have the specific factors underpinning this symbiosis been identified. Nutrition covers a spectrum from general host nutrition to specific supplements and micronutrients. All aspects of nutrition within this spectrum contribute to the wound healing process. Likewise, deficits or absence of certain components of nutrition can be detrimental to healing. This article explores the role of nutrition in wound healing and summarizes much of the current literature regarding nutritional supplementation and pharmacologic modulation of the wound healing process.

Converging and replicated evidence indicates that psychological stress can modulate wound-healing processes. This article reviews the methods and findings of experimental models of wound healing. Psychological stress can have a substantial and clinically relevant impact on wound repair. Physiologic stress responses can directly influence wound-healing processes. Furthermore, psychological stress can indirectly modulate the repair process by promoting the adoption of health-damaging behaviors. Translational work is needed to develop innovative treatments able to attenuate stress-induced delays in wound healing.

> This article focuses primarily on the recent literature on abdominal compartment syndrome (ACS) and the definitions and recommendations published by the World Society for the Abdominal Compartment Syndrome. The definitions regarding increased intra-abdominal pressure (IAP) are listed and are followed by an overview of the different mechanisms of organ dysfunction associated with intra-abdominal hypertension (IAH). Measurement techniques for IAP are discussed, as are recommendations for organ function support and options for treatment in patients who have IAH. ACS was first described in surgical patients who had abdominal trauma, bleeding, or infection; but recently, ACS has been described in patients who have other pathologies. This article intends to provide critical care physicians with a clear insight into the current state of knowledge regarding IAH and ACS.

> Compartment syndrome should be treated early and aggressively to prevent late complications. Patients may have late deformity because of a failure of diagnosis, inadequate decompression, or a delay in fasciotomies. Late reconstruction will allow a plantigrade and relatively functional foot. Complete excision of scarred muscle will prevent recurrence in established deformities. Early treatment may prevent significant functional impairment by well-placed tenotomies. In patients with severe long-term deformities with extensive soft tissue contraction, incremental correction may be an appropriate intermediate intervention.

> Postoperative infections continue to be a challenging problem. The incidence of bacterial antibiotic resistance such as methicillin-resistant Staphylococcus aureus is rising. There are numerous intrinsic patient factors that should be optimized before surgery to minimize the risk of surgical site infections. When postoperative infections develop, treatment must be individualized. This article outlines the principles that can help guide treatment.

CRITICAL CARE NURSING CLINICS

Preface

Many critically ill patients have complex wounds that are challenging to manage and consume extensive resources in supplies, personnel time, prolonged lengths of stay, and monetary costs. A majority of wounds arise from clean case surgeries, with an estimated 30 million procedures annually in the United States, with 3% to 4% complicated by infection.[1] Organ transplantation, delicate reconstructive surgery, and complex orthopedic surgeries are examples of procedures that may necessitate care in the intensive care unit. The picture worsens for patients with traumatic injuries and other wounds, with greater infection rates in wounds sustained in uncontrolled environments. Examples include blunt and sharp traumatic injuries, blast injuries, burns, and fractures. Compartment syndrome is a complication that can occur in both upper and lower extremities and the abdomen and may follow orthopedic surgery and a variety of traumatic injuries. Preexisting medical conditions such as diabetes mellitus and peripheral vascular disease may generate the wound or they can complicate healing of wounds from other sources. Additional characteristics of critical illness such as insufficient nutrition and hydration, immobility, and vasopressor use aggravate the healing process. This can lead to problems such as extreme and prolonged pain, deconditioning, disability, and disfigurement.

This issue begins with a detailed description of the phases of wound healing (Goldberg and Diegelman) and guidelines for facilitating the process. Williams and Barbul describe the impact of nutrition on wound healing. They discuss the role of carbohydrates, fats, amino acids, vitamins, and minerals, along with the benefits and risks of total parenteral nutrition. In the fascinating article by Gouin and Kiecolt-Glaser, the psychological effects of wound healing are discussed. They address the neurohormonal response to stress and the impediment to tissue repair.

Wound management is the focus of the next three articles. Moreira and Markovchick provide an emergency provider's clinical approach to include guidance during the history and physical exam, diagnostic studies, and wound-closure methods specific for injuries to various bodily structures. In the article by Beitz, the indications for and types of debridement are discussed, including surgical, mechanical, chemical, autolytic, enzymatic, biotherapeutic, and laser methods. Finally, Adams, Sabesan, and Easley summarize the available wound-healing agents, including various dressing types and adjuvant therapy such as vacuum assistance and hyperbaric therapy.

In the next three articles, the challenges of compartment syndrome-related wounds are discussed. Friedrich and Shin focus on the forearm. They apply the pathophysiological concepts of compartment syndrome to the anatomical structures, with a description of the surgical transfer and repair of tendons, muscle, and fascia. In the article by Malbrain and De laet an extensive description of the pathophysiology of compartment syndrome is provided, with application to the thoracic, abdominal, and retroperitoneal organs. A description of surgical decompression, open abdominal wound, and systemic treatment is provided. Lastly, Perry and Manoli describe the surgical management for early treatment as well as late deformities of the foot sustained by leg or foot compartment syndrome.

Crit Care Nurs Clin N Am 24 (2012) ix–x
doi:10.1016/j.ccell.2012.03.011
0899-5885/12/$ – see front matter © 2012 Elsevier Inc. All rights reserved.

ccnursing.theclinics.com

The issue concludes with an article by Gaston and Kuremsky concerning prevention and management of postoperative infections. Preventive measures include preoperative modifiable and nonmodifiable risk factors; skin preparation and hair removal; and intraoperative risk factors. Management approaches discussed include antimicrobial therapy and wound vacuum. The authors provide recommendations for special postoperative infections including septic arthritis, osteomyelitis, and necrotizing fasciitis.

Jan Foster, PhD, APRN, CNS, CCRN
Nursing Inquiry and Intervention, Inc.
58 Aberdeen Crossing
The Woodlands, TX 77381, USA
Texas Woman's University
6400 Fannin Houston,
TX 77030, USA

E-mail address:
jfoster@twu.edu

REFERENCE

1. Wenzel RP. Minimizing surgical-site infections. N Engl J Med 2010;362:75–7.

Wound Healing Primer

Stephanie R. Goldberg, MD[a], Robert F. Diegelmann, PhD[b],*

KEYWORDS

- Acute wound • Phases of healing • Healing mechanisms • Guidelines for healing

KEY POINTS

- The healing of surgical, acute, and chronic wounds requires the complex interaction of a multitude of cells, growth factors, and other proteins to allow the return of structure and function.
- Wound healing research only continues to evolve. With the creation of the Wound Healing Society guidelines as well as the significant contributions from researchers studying wound healing, the ability to modulate nonhealing wounds and facilitate wound closure continues to improve.

Surgeons often care for patients with conditions of abnormal wound healing, which include conditions of excessive wound healing, such as fibrosis, adhesions, and contractures, as well as conditions of inadequate wound healing, such as chronic nonhealing ulcers, recurrent hernias, and wound dehiscences. Despite many recent advances in the field, which have highlighted the importance of adjunct therapies in maximizing the healing potential, such as optimization of nutrition, growth factor therapy, advanced wound dressing materials, and bioengineered skin substitutes, conditions of abnormal wound healing continue to cause significant cost, morbidity, and mortality. To understand how conditions of abnormal wound healing can be corrected, it is important to first understand the basic principles of wound healing.

PHASES OF WOUND HEALING

Wound healing consists of a complex but very orderly array of overlapping phases in which highly specialized cells interact with an extracellular matrix to lay down a new framework for tissue growth and repair.[1] There are 4 distinct but overlapping phases of wound healing, which include hemostasis, inflammation, proliferation, and remodeling (**Fig. 1**). These phases are influenced by the various cellular interactions and are

A version of this article was previously published in *Surgical Clinics* 90:6.

[a] Department of Surgery, Virginia Commonwealth University Medical Center, West Hospital, 16th Floor, West Wing, 1200 East Broad Street, Richmond, VA 23298-0645, USA; [b] Department of Biochemistry and Molecular Biology, Virginia Commonwealth University Medical Center, 1101 East Marshall Street, Sanger Hall, Room 2-007, Richmond, VA 23298-0614, USA
* Corresponding author.
E-mail address: rdiegelm@vcu.edu

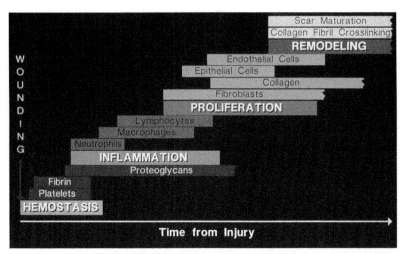

Fig. 1. Phases of normal wound healing. Cellular and molecular events during normal wound healing progress through 4 major integrated phases: hemostasis, inflammation, proliferation, and remodeling. (*From* Cohen IK, Diegelmann RF, Lindblad WJ, editors. Wound healing: biochemical and clinical aspects. Philadelphia: W.B. Saunders; 1993; with permission.)

regulated by the local release of chemical signals such as cytokines, chemokines, growth factors, and inhibitors.[2,3]

HEMOSTASIS PHASE

Immediately after tissue injury, hemostasis occurs to minimize hemorrhage. While the blood vessels constrict, platelets are activated by binding to the exposed collagen in the extracellular matrix. The platelets then release fibronectin, thrombospondin, sphingosine 1 phosphate, and von Willebrand factor, which promote further platelet activation and aggregation.[4] As these activation and other clotting factors are released, a fibrin matrix is deposited in the wound, which functions as a provisional matrix to stabilize the wound site. The aggregated platelets then become trapped in the fibrin matrix, thus forming a stable clot within the provisional matrix (**Fig. 2**).[5]

Several important mediators that are released by platelets are responsible for the initiation and progression of wounds through the subsequent phases of wound healing. These mediators include platelet-derived growth factor (PDGF) and transforming growth factor β (TGF-β). TGF-β and PDGF recruit additional cells, such as neutrophils and macrophages, to enter the wound. PDGF also recruits fibroblasts to the wound and activates the production of collagen and glycosaminoglycans by fibroblasts, which are important for the repair of the extracellular matrix.[2,3,6] Excessive levels of these growth factors have been indicated in conditions of abnormal wound healing; TGF-β is also present in many fibrotic conditions such as pulmonary fibrosis and cirrhosis.[7,8]

INFLAMMATORY PHASE

The next phase of wound healing is inflammation, which begins within the first 24 hours after an injury. The stage can last up to 2 weeks in patients whose wounds are healing appropriately but can last longer in those patients with chronic nonhealing wounds. From a clinical standpoint, this stage is characterized by rubor (redness),

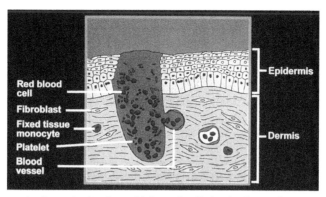

Fig. 2. Hemostasis phase. At the time of injury, the fibrin clot forms the provisional wound matrix and platelets release multiple growth factors that initiate the repair process. (*From* Greenfield LJ, editor. Surgery: scientific principles and practice. Philadelphia: J.B. Lippincott, 1993; with permission.)

calor (heat), tumor (swelling), and dolor (pain), which results from the release of vasoactive amines and histamine-rich granules from the mast cells. These mast cell mediators cause surrounding vessels to become leaky and thus allow the efficient movement of neutrophils from the vasculature to the site of injury. Because the vessels become leaky, fluid also escapes into the area and thus causes the swelling (tumor) and pressure-causing pain (dolor).

In addition to mast cells, neutrophils and macrophages play key roles in the inflammatory phase (**Fig. 3**). Neutrophils serve as a first line of defense against infection by phagocytosing bacteria, damaged extracellular components, and foreign materials. As various chemical signals are released from the wound site, the

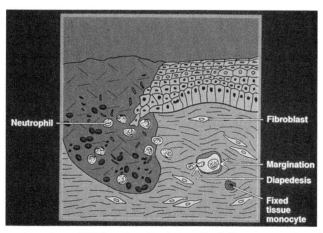

Fig. 3. Inflammatory phase. Within a day after injury, the inflammatory phase is initiated by neutrophils that attach to endothelial cells in the vessel walls surrounding the wound (margination), change shape and move through the cell junctions (diapedesis), and migrate to the wound site (chemotaxis). (*From* Greenfield LJ, editor. Surgery: scientific principles and practice. Philadelphia: J.B. Lippincott, 1993; with permission.)

endothelial cells in the nearby vessels are activated and begin to express specialized cell adhesion molecules (CAMs) called selectins. These CAMs function as molecular hooks to grab circulating neutrophils to bind to the endothelial cell surface by a process called pavementing. The adherent neutrophils begin to roll along the endothelial cell lining and then by a process called diapedesis, they squeeze through the cell junctions that have been made leaky by the mast cell mediators.[9,10]

The neutrophils are attracted to the site of injury by a process called chemotaxis and are drawn there by soluble mediators, such as a breakdown product of a complement called C5a, a tripeptide f-Met-Leu-Phe (N-formyl-methionyl-leucyl-phenylalanine) that is a waste product produced by bacteria that may be present in the wound, and the potent chemokine interleukin (IL)-8.[11–13] To move through the extracellular matrix, the neutrophils release matrix-degrading enzymes, such as elastase and matrix metalloproteinase (MMP)-8, a collagenase. During a normal acute wound healing response, these enzymes are released in physiologic amounts and do not cause excessive tissue damage. In contrast, in many nonhealing chronic wounds, there is an overabundance of neutrophils, releasing massive amounts of these matrix-destroying enzymes that cause excessive damage to the extracellular matrix as well as the destruction of critical growth factors such as PDGF and TGF-β.[14–16] These ulcers are locked into a continuous inflammatory phase, resulting in extensive loss of tissue.[17]

On their arrival at the wound site, the neutrophils begin to aggressively phagocytize any foreign materials and kill bacteria by the powerful battery of enzymes and reactive oxygen species, which they can generate. The neutrophils actually initiate the first stages of the proliferative phase by releasing IL-1 and tumor necrosis factor (TNF)-α to begin the activation of fibroblasts and epithelial cells.

During the inflammatory phase, activated wound macrophages also play a key role in the regulation and progression of wound healing. Wound macrophages are derived from fixed tissue monocytes that originate from circulating monocytes (see **Fig. 3**). The wound macrophages are activated by chemokines, cytokines, growth factors, and soluble fragments of extracellular matrix components produced by proteolytic degradation of collagen and fibronectin.[18] The wound macrophages function to remove any residual bacteria, foreign bodies, and remaining necrotic tissue. The function of these macrophages is therefore similar to that of neutrophils, but macrophages better regulate proteolytic destruction of wound tissue by secreting protease inhibitors. In addition, macrophages ingest the bacteria-laden neutrophils and mediate progression of the wound from the inflammatory to the proliferative phase. Macrophages also secrete a multitude of growth factors and cytokines, such as PDGF, TGF-β, TNF-α, fibroblast growth factor (FGF), insulinlike growth factor 1, and IL-6, which then recruit fibroblasts and endothelial cells to the wound site for matrix deposition and neovascularization.

PROLIFERATIVE PHASE

The proliferative phase is characterized by fibroblast proliferation and collagen deposition to replace the provisional fibrin matrix and to provide a stable extracellular matrix at the wound site. The new matrix consists of collagen, proteoglycans, and fibronectins. In addition, angiogenesis occurs such that new blood vessels replace the previously damaged capillaries and provide nourishment for the matrix. Granulation tissue formation and the process of epithelization also occur.

Fibroblasts migrate into the wound in response to mediators released from the platelets and macrophages and move through the extracellular matrix by binding fibronectin, vitronectin, and fibrin via their RGD or arginine-glycine-aspartic acid

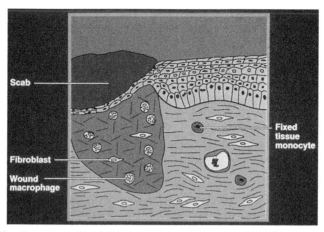

Fig. 4. Proliferation phase. Fixed tissue monocytes become activated, move into the site of injury, transform into activated wound macrophages that kill bacteria, release proteases that remove denatured extracellular matrix, and secrete growth factors that stimulate fibroblast, epidermal cells, and endothelial cells to proliferate and produce scar tissue. (*From* Greenfield LJ, editor. Surgery: scientific principles and practice. Philadelphia: J.B. Lippincott, 1993; with permission.)

amino acid sequence recognized by their integrin receptors (**Fig. 4**). The fibroblasts also secrete MMPs, which facilitate their movement through the matrix and help with the removal of damaged matrix components. Once the fibroblasts have entered the wound, they produce collagen, proteoglycans, and other components. Fibroblast activity is predominately regulated by PDGF and TGF-β. PDGF, secreted by platelets and macrophages, stimulates fibroblast proliferation, chemotaxis, and collagenase expression.

TGF-β has a central role in wound healing. There are 3 isoforms of TGF-β, which include TGF-β1, TGF-β2, and TGF-β3. TGF-β1 has been found to be present in excess amounts in conditions of fibrosis, such as pulmonary fibrosis and cirrhosis.[7,8] Although little is known about TGF-β2, TGF-β3 is associated with a reduction in fibrosis and scarring.[19] Despite their opposite effects on fibrosis, TGF-β2 and TGF-β3 bind the same TGF-β type 2 seronine/threonine kinase receptor, which then joins together with a TGF-β receptor (TBR) type 1 to activate the Smad cell signaling pathways.[20] Thus, activation of signaling cascades by the various TGF-β isoforms may account for the presence or lack of fibrosis within the wounds.

The most convincing studies that suggest a role for TGF-β in wound healing have been done in fetal animal models. Fetal mouse incisional wounds are known to heal without scarring and with a negligible amount of TGF-β present.[21,22] Lanning and colleagues[23] report that midgestational fetal wounds in the rabbit can be stimulated to contract in the presence of TGF-β1 and TGF-β3. In a study on the fetal mouse, rapid midgestational wound closure was associated with an increase in TGF-β1 and TBR-2 expressions compared with surrounding normal skin.[24]

Endothelial cells are activated by TNF-α and basic FGF (bFGF) to initiate angiogenesis such that new blood vessels are initiated to promote blood flow to support the high metabolic activity in the newly deposited tissue. Angiogenesis is regulated by a combination of local stimulatory factors, such as vascular endothelial cell growth factor (VEGF), and antiangiogenic factors, such as angiostatin, endostatin, thrombospondin, and pigment epithelium-derived growth factor. Local factors that stimulate angiogenesis include low oxygen tension, low pH, and high lactate levels.[25] Oxygen-sensing proteins regulate the transcription of angiogenic and antiangiogenic genes. Soluble mediators, such as bFGF, TGF-β, and VEGF, also stimulate endothelial cells to produce blood vessels. Tissue oxygen levels directly regulate angiogenesis through hypoxia inducible factor (HIF), which binds oxygen.[26] When there is a decrease in oxygen levels surrounding capillary endothelial cells, HIF-1 levels increase inside the cells and HIF-1 binds to specific DNA sequences to stimulate VEGF transcription to promote angiogenesis.

As the wound continues to heal, the granulation tissue forms to provide the transitional replacement for normal dermis and ultimately evolves into a scar. Granulation tissue consists of a dense network of blood vessels and capillaries, elevated cellular density of fibroblasts and macrophages, and randomly organized collagen fibers. The metabolic rate is also higher for this tissue compared with normal dermis, which reflects the activity required for cellular migration, division, and protein synthesis and thus, the importance of adequate nutrition and oxygen to properly heal the wound.

REMODELING PHASE

The last phase of wound healing is the remodeling phase in which granulation tissue matures into a scar (**Fig. 5**). Small capillaries aggregate into larger blood vessels and there is an overall decrease in the water content of the wound. Similarly, cell density and overall metabolic activity of the wound decrease. Perhaps the most dramatic change occurs in the overall type, amount, and organization of collagen fibers, resulting in increased tensile strength of the wound. Initially, there is increased deposition of type III collagen, also referred to as reticular collagen, that is gradually replaced by type I collagen, the dominant fibrillar collagen in skin.[27] Collagen fibers are cross-linked by the enzyme lysyl oxidase, which is secreted by fibroblasts in the extracellular matrix. As the wound continues to remodel, changes in collagen

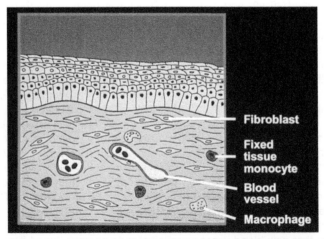

Fig. 5. Remodeling phase. The initial disorganized scar tissue is slowly replaced by a matrix that more closely resembles the organized extracellular matrix of normal skin. (*From* Greenfield LJ, editor. Surgery: scientific principles and practice. Philadelphia: J.B. Lippincott, 1993; with permission.)

organization increases the tensile strength to a maximum of about 80% of normal tissue.

Extracellular zinc-dependent endopeptidases called MMPs have recently emerged as an exciting area in wound healing, which may have promising therapeutic potential. MMPs control the degradation of extracellular matrix components to facilitate epithelial cell migration into the wound, angiogenesis, and overall tissue remodeling. MMPs are secreted by epidermal cells and modulate tissue inhibitors of metallopro-teinases (TIMPs) as well as degrade other growth factors.[28–31] Low levels of MMPs are found in normal tissue but increased levels of MMP-1 and MMP-2 are present in keloids, a condition of excess collagen deposition after cutaneous injury.[32] Similarly, a disruption in the balance between MMPs and their inhibitors has been reported in diabetic and venous stasis ulcers.[33,34] In addition, MMPs can be found in increased levels in chronic wounds.[35–38] Yager and colleagues[39] report that there are more than 10-fold higher levels of MMP-2 and 25-fold higher levels of MMP-9 in fluid from pressure ulcers compared with surgical wounds.

MMP expression is regulated by TGF-β. In normal fibroblasts and keratinocytes, abrogation of TGF-β1 is associated with decreased levels of MMPs and increased angiogenesis.[40–42] Tissue samples from keloids have demonstrated increased levels of MMP-2 and MMP-9 compared with healthy skin. Abrogation of TGF-β1 in keloid-derived fibroblasts results in a downregulation of MMP-9, further demonstrat-ing the important relationship between TGF-β and MMPs.[43]

Treatment strategies targeted at the control of excess MMPs in chronic wounds have included the use of protease inhibitors to decrease MMP levels in the wounds and surrounding tissue. Oral and topical doxycycline, a potent MMP inhibitor, has been shown to decrease inflammation and matrix destruction.[44] Further studies are necessary to determine the clinical efficacy of doxycycline and other MMP inhibitors on chronic wounds.[45] TGF-β also minimizes matrix degradation by downregulating protease secretion and stimulating synthesis of TIMP.

As the extracellular matrix continues to remodel, collagen synthesis and degrada-tion are ongoing as the matrix strives to achieve the original highly organized structure that was present before the wound injury. The scar tissue is always weaker than the normal surrounding matrix and can only achieve about 80% of the tensile strength that was present initially. If degradation maintains an equilibrium, then a fine line scar forms. If matrix synthesis is greater than degradation, then a hypertrophic scar may form. Conversely, if matrix degradation is greater than synthesis or if synthesis is inhibited by pharmacologic agents, such as steroids or cancer chemotherapeutic agents, or perhaps by malnutrition, the scar becomes too weak and wound dehis-cence can occur.

MECHANISMS OF WOUND HEALING

Dermal wounds heal by 3 main mechanisms: connective tissue deposition, contrac-tion, and epithelialization. Depending on the type of wound, these 3 distinct processes come into play to varying degrees. For example, an acute linear wound, such as a surgical incision that is closed by the surgeon using sutures, staples, tapes, or perhaps dermal glue, heals by what is termed primary intention. The major mechanism needed to heal wounds by primary intention is the process of connective tissue deposition. No contraction is needed because the surgeon has closed the incision by mechanical means. There is only minimal epithelization, which occurs along the wound line on the surface.

Open wounds, in which there is a loss of tissue, such as seen when a fingertip is injured, heal by a process termed secondary intention. These open wounds heal mainly by tissue contraction in which a centripetal force is generated by an interaction between fibroblasts and the matrix to advance the edges toward the center of the wound. There maybe some matrix deposition, and what is not achieved by those 2 processes is then covered by epithelization. Some chronic wounds, such as pressure ulcers, also heal by secondary intention once the chronic inflammation is controlled and granulation tissue is allowed to form.

If an open wound is suspected to be contaminated with foreign debris or bacteria, then the wound must be kept open and treated with gentle irrigation until the foreign materials and infectious agents are removed. As a general guide, the total bacterial burden should be lower than 10^5 organisms/g of tissue, as determined by biopsy and culturing.[46] Surface swabs are generally thought to be inaccurate. The wound should be gently irrigated with saline or lactated Ringer, and pressures greater than 15 psi should be avoided because they can force materials deeper into the wound bed and also damage newly forming granulation tissue.[47] Once these goals are achieved and if the wound can be closed, then the wound heals by a mechanism termed delayed primary intention.

Epithelialization is the process whereby epithelial cells surrounding the wound margin or in residual skin appendages, such as rete pegs, hair follicles, and sebaceous glands, migrate into the wound because of the loss of contact inhibition of cuboidal basal keratinocytes.[48] This type of healing is termed partial thickness healing and is observed in minor abrasions and skin graft donor sites when an approximately 0.015 in thick piece of skin is removed for coverage elsewhere on the patient. After an extensive multistep process, these basal epithelial cells proliferate near the wound margin, producing a monolayer that moves over the wound surface.

DEFINITION OF WOUNDS

For many years, lack of uniform definitions in the generalized description of wounds served as an impediment in setting forth guidelines for the treatment of wounds. In 1994, the Wound Healing Society sought to standardize the definitions of wounds and the evaluation of wound healing. A wound is defined as a disruption in the normal anatomic structure and function. Wounds can be classified as acute or chronic based on whether or not they progress through an orderly and timely healing process so as to restore anatomic continuity and function. Wounds are further differentiated based according to whether they are ideally healed, minimally healed, or acceptably healed based on various degrees of restoration of normal anatomy, function, structure, and appearance.[49] The problems associated with diabetic venous stasis and other complex and difficult wounds are addressed elsewhere in this issue.

GUIDELINES FOR THE HEALING OF ACUTE WOUNDS

The Wound Healing Society identified 11 categories of impediment to wound healing to formulate guidelines to promote the healing of acute wounds.[50] These include local impediments such as wound perfusion, tissue viability, hematoma and/or seroma, infection, and mechanical factors as well as systemic impediments that include immunologic factors, oncologic factors, miscellaneous systemic conditions, thermal injuries, external agents, and excessive scarring. The following summarizes the main clinical recommendations of the published guidelines.

Adequate blood supply must exist to provide oxygenation and nourishment to healing wounds, which can be maximized for elective surgical wounds by ruling out clinically significant arterial disease by the presence of palpable pulses or ankle-brachial indexes greater than 0.9, calculated as the ratio of the resting systolic pressure in the arteries of the ankle to that of the brachial artery. The lack of sufficient blood supply may lead to tissue ischemia and an increased risk of infection. Similarly, hypotension in the setting of acute wounds should be minimized. Patients should be advised to avoid smoking, blood glucose levels should be controlled, and hypothermia should be avoided, so to further maximize blood flow to the wounds.[51] The use of supplemental hyperbaric oxygen has long been thought to augment wound healing by increasing tissue oxygen levels; however, it has varied usage in the clinical setting. The Wound Healing Society guidelines suggest that more clinical data are necessary to support its use in acute wounds; however, a recent study demonstrated improved wound tissue oxygen tension in obese patients with supplemental oxygen administration.[52]

Wounds must be debrided of devitalized and infected tissue by one of the following methods, including preferably sharp surgical debridement and also enzymatic, mechanical, biologic or autolytic therapies. The formation of fluid collections, including hematomas, should be minimized by meticulous control of intraoperative hemostasis and correction of preoperative coagulopathies. Heparin prophylaxis against venous thromboembolism is indicated but may increase bleeding complications. There is no evidence according to the Wound Healing Society guidelines that antiplatelet agents increase the risk of hematomas. Similarly, the formation of seromas in patients with large skin flaps (mastectomy or component separation) should be minimized by closure of dead space and placement of surgical drains. The accumulation of fluid and blood may lead to local ischemia, necrosis, and an infected wound. Thus, postoperative fluid collections should be drained either surgically or percutaneously when possible.

Wounds should not be primarily closed if there is more than 10^5 bacteria/g of tissue or any amount of β-hemolytic streptococci because of an increased risk of wound infection.[46] A single dose of preoperative antibiotics is an indication in clean-contaminated or contaminated cases. Preoperative antibiotics are only recommended in clean cases if prosthetic materials, such as mesh, are implanted. Prophylactic antibiotics are not indicated in superficial nonbite injuries but should be used in bite injuries from animals and humans because they result in wound contamination. The risk of surgical site infections can further be decreased with normothermia and avoidance of hypoxia. Preoperative shaving of hair or scrubbing of the skin is not necessary to decrease the risk of infection because the bacterial load of normal skin flora is in the range of 10^3 organisms/g of tissue.

Wounds heal faster when closed primarily than those left to heal by secondary intention. Wounds should, however, be closed in a tension-free manner. Laparotomy incisions should be closed in a continuous manner using a suture length to wound length ratio of 4:1. The suture material used should be present until adequate tensile strength is obtained. The specific type of suture material used is irrelevant; however, permanent sutures are associated with an increased risk of fistulization. In patients with open abdomens, distractive forces that minimize subsequent fascial closure may be minimized through the use of negative pressure therapy. Retention sutures, long thought to be useful in preventing fascial dehiscence, do not prevent breakdown of the abdominal wall incisions.

Systemic immune defenses in patients with immune deficiencies should be maximized with the use of prophylaxis antibiotics, especially in patients with conditions such as AIDS. When possible, patients on immunosuppressants or steroid drugs should be weaned to the lowest possible dose preoperatively. Blood transfusions should be used with caution because they may result in transient immunosuppression.[53] Granulocyte-macrophage colony-stimulating growth factor may be used to correct leukopenia preoperatively so as to further maximize wound healing, but definitive studies have not been done to date.[54] In patients with cancer, operation performed through nonradiated tissue planes is associated with improved outcomes in wound healing. In addition, good nutrition is essential for optimal wound healing and can be augmented using preferably enteral means. Good nutrition is especially important in elderly patients and in those with cancer. Nutrition has traditionally been assessed by the measurement of prealbumin; however, this marker has proved to be unreliable in conditions of inflammation, acute renal failure, and corticosteroid use,[55] There are also insufficient data to support exogenous use of vitamins unless there is clear documentation of specific nutrient deficiencies such as those of vitamin C.

Burn injuries can be characterized as complex wounds consisting of shallow-partial thickness wounds, deep wounds, donor-site wounds resulting from skin graft harvest, or interstitial wounds from skin grafts. Each type of wound requires a different type of treatment. Partial-thickness wounds typically epithelialize within 21 days, whereas deeper wounds may require debridement of necrotic tissue with subsequent skin grafting for tissue coverage. Early debridement of deep burns has been advocated to minimize infection risk from necrotic tissue and promote normal healing, which has been associated with improved survivals. Permanent skin substitutes or temporary biologic or biosynthetic dressings may be used as an alternative to skin grafting should the excited burn total body surface area be too large to allow for donor grating. Deep wounds that cannot undergo early debridement may benefit from topical antibacterial agents; however, these agents have not been shown to be beneficial on shallow wounds, donor sites, or meshed skin grafts. There is no role for systemically administered antibiotics in the absence of systemic infection. The role of various vitamins and cofactors to augment wound healing is controversial. Zinc therapy may improve wound healing in zinc-deficient patients, yet routine use of zinc is not indicated. There are insufficient data to support the definitive use of vitamin C, vitamin E, and arginine. Pressure garments or compression dressings may be used to decrease fibrosis and scarring in burn injuries requiring more than 21 days to heal. Proliferative scars may benefit from silicone sheeting to decrease fibroblast activity and downregulate TGF-β. Direct injection of corticosteroids, including triamcinolone acetonide (Kenalog), may also improve proliferative scars. Postoperative radiation for benign conditions must be used with extreme caution; however, laser therapy may be useful.

Improved healing has not been seen in children or elderly with scald burns as well as in those with either inhalation injury or burns to the face and hands.

NORMAL AND PATHOLOGIC RESPONSES TO WOUND HEALING

Acute wounds progress through the phases in an orderly fashion for normal healing to occur. Chronic wounds begin the healing process in a similar fashion; however, they have prolonged inflammatory phase in which there is significant destruction of the matrix elements caused by the release of proteolytic enzymes from the neutrophils.[14–17] Once the excessive inflammation is controlled by aggressive wound care, then the proliferative and remodeling phases begin; however, the resulting scar is often excessive and fibrotic.[56] These chronic nonhealing ulcers are examples of severely deficient healing and are addressed in detail elsewhere in this issue. Despite extensive research into the mechanisms underlying wound healing, patients continue to be plagued by such pathologic conditions of abnormal wound healing in other tissues and organs, including recurrent and incisional hernias, anastomotic leaks, and wound dehiscence.

In conditions of fibrosis, the equilibrium between scar deposition and remodeling is such that an excessive amount of collagen deposition and organization occurs. This condition leads to a loss of both structure and function. Fibrosis, strictures, adhesions, keloids, hypertrophic scars, and contractures are examples of excessive pathologic healing.

Clinical differences between chronic and acute healing wounds are thought to be, in part, explained by alterations in the local biochemical environment. Acute wounds are associated with a greater mitogenic activity than chronic wounds.[57–59] Chronic wounds are associated with a higher level of proinflammatory cytokines than acute wounds. As chronic wounds begin to heal, they progress to a less proinflammatory state. Chronic wounds have elevated levels of MMPs compared with acute wounds.[16,39,56,60] Elevated protease activities in some chronic wounds may directly contribute to poor healing by degrading proteins necessary for normal wound healing, such as extracellular matrix proteins, growth factors, and protease inhibitors. Steed and colleagues[61] reported that extensive debridement of diabetic ulcers resulted in improved healing in patients treated with placebo or with recombinant human PDGF. Frequent debridement may therefore allow a chronic wound to heal in a similar fashion to an acute wound. In addition to the local wound environment, there are data to suggest that cells of chronic wounds may have an altered capacity by which to respond to various cytokines and growth factors and are in a senescent state.[62]

SUMMARY

The healing of surgical, acute, and chronic wounds requires the complex interaction of a multitude of cells, growth factors, and other proteins to allow the return of structure and function. Wound healing research only continues to evolve. With the creation of the Wound Healing Society guidelines as well as the significant contributions from researchers studying wound healing, the ability to modulate nonhealing wounds and facilitate wound closure continues to improve (http://www.woundheal.org).

REFERENCES

1. Diegelmann RF, Evans MC. Wound healing: an overview of acute, fibrotic and delayed healing. Front Biosci 2004;9:283–9.
2. Bennett NT, Schultz GS. Growth factors and wound healing: part II. Role in normal and chronic wound healing. Am J Surg 1993;166(1):74–81.
3. Bennett NT, Schultz GS. Growth factors and wound healing: biochemical properties of growth factors and their receptors. Am J Surg 1993;165(6):728–37.
4. Cho J, Mosher DF. Role of fibronectin assembly in platelet thrombus formation. J Thromb Haemost 2006;4(7):1461–9.
5. Gailit J, Clark RA. Wound repair in the context of extracellular matrix. Curr Opin Cell Biol 1994;6(5):717–25.
6. Rumalla VK, Borah GL. Cytokines, growth factors, and plastic surgery. Plast Reconstr Surg 2001;108(3):719–33.
7. Broekelmann TJ, Limper AH, Colby TV, et al. Transforming growth factor beta 1 is present at sites of extracellular matrix gene expression in human pulmonary fibrosis. Proc Natl Acad Sci U S A 1991;88(15):6642–6.
8. Gressner AM, Weiskirchen R, Breitkopf K, et al. Roles of TGF-beta in hepatic fibrosis. Front Biosci 2002;7:d793–807.
9. Frenette PS, Wagner DD. Adhesion molecules—part 1. N Engl J Med 1996;334(23):1526–9.
10. Frenette PS, Wagner DD. Adhesion molecules—part II: blood vessels and blood cells. N Engl J Med 1996;335(1):43–5.
11. Guo RF, Ward PA. Role of C5a in inflammatory responses. Annu Rev Immunol 2005;23:821–52.

12. Tschaikowsky K, Sittl R, Braun GG, et al. Increased fMet-Leu-Phe receptor expression and altered superoxide production of neutrophil granulocytes in septic and posttraumatic patients. Clin Investig 1993;72(1):18–25.

13. Roupe KM, Nybo M, Sjobring U, et al. Injury is a major inducer of epidermal innate immune responses during wound healing. J Invest Dermatol 2010;130(4):1167–77.

14. Nwomeh BC, Liang HX, Cohen IK, et al. MMP-8 is the predominant collagenase in healing wounds and nonhealing ulcers. J Surg Res 1999;81(2):189–95.

15. Nwomeh BC, Liang HX, Diegelmann RF, et al. Dynamics of the matrix metalloproteinases MMP-1 and MMP-8 in acute open human dermal wounds. Wound Repair Regen 1998;6(2):127–34.

16. Yager DR, Chen SM, Ward S, et al. The ability of chronic wound fluids to degrade peptide growth factors is associated with increased levels of elastase activity and diminished levels of proteinase inhibitors. Wound Repair Regen 1997;5:23–32.

17. Diegelmann RF. Excessive neutrophils characterize chronic pressure ulcers. Wound Repair Regen 2003;11(6):490–5.

18. Diegelmann RF, Cohen IK, Kaplan AM. The role of macrophages in wound repair: a review. Plast Reconstr Surg 1981;68(1):107–13.

19. Shah M, Foreman DM, Ferguson MW. Neutralisation of TGF-beta 1 and TGF-beta 2 or exogenous addition of TGF-beta 3 to cutaneous rat wounds reduces scarring. J Cell Sci 1995;108(Pt 3):985–1002.

20. ten Dijke P, Hill CS. New insights into TGF-beta-Smad signaling. Trends Biochem Sci 2004;29(5):265–73.

21. Stelnicki EJ, Bullard KM, Harrison MR, et al. A new in vivo model for the study of fetal wound healing. Ann Plast Surg 1997;39(4):374–80.

22. Whitby DJ, Ferguson MW. Immunohistochemical localization of growth factors in fetal wound healing. Dev Biol 1991;147(1):207–15.

23. Lanning DA, Nwomeh BC, Montante SJ, et al. TGF-beta1 alters the healing of cutaneous fetal excisional wounds. J Pediatr Surg 1999;34(5):695–700.

24. Goldberg SR, McKinstry RP, Sykes V, et al. Rapid closure of midgestational excisional wounds in a fetal mouse model is associated with altered transforming growth factor-beta isoform and receptor expression. J Pediatr Surg 2007;42(6):966–71 [discussion: 971–3].

25. Bhushan M, Young HS, Brenchley PE, et al. Recent advances in cutaneous angiogenesis. Br J Dermatol 2002;147(3):418–25.

26. Semenza GL. HIF-1 and tumor progression: pathophysiology and therapeutics. Trends Mol Med 2002;8(Suppl 4):S62–7.

27. Clore JN, Cohen IK, Diegelmann RF. Quantitation of collagen types I and III during wound healing in rat skin. Proc Soc Exp Biol Med 1979;161(3):337–40.

28. Chen WY, Rogers AA, Lydon MJ. Characterization of biologic properties of wound fluid collected during early stages of wound healing. J Invest Dermatol 1992;99(5):559–64.

29. Vaalamo M, Leivo T, Saarialho-Kere U. Differential expression of tissue inhibitors of metalloproteinases (TIMP-1, -2, -3, and -4) in normal and aberrant wound healing. Hum Pathol 1999;30(7):795–802.

30. Trengove NJ, Stacey MC, MacAuley S, et al. Analysis of the acute and chronic wound environments: the role of proteases and their inhibitors. Wound Repair Regen 1999;7(6):442–52.

31. Singer AJ, Clark RA. Cutaneous wound healing. N Engl J Med 1999;341(10):738–46.

32. Thielitz A, Vetter RW, Schultze B, et al. Inhibitors of dipeptidyl peptidase IV-like activity mediate antifibrotic effects in normal and keloid-derived skin fibroblasts. J Invest Dermatol 2008;128(4):855–66.

33. Cowin AJ, Hatzirodos N, Holding CA, et al. Effect of healing on the expression of transforming growth factor beta(s) and their receptors in chronic venous leg ulcers. J Invest Dermatol 2001;117(5):1282–9.
34. Galkowska H, Wojewodzka U, Olszewski WL. Chemokines, cytokines, and growth factors in keratinocytes and dermal endothelial cells in the margin of chronic diabetic foot ulcers. Wound Repair Regen 2006;14(5):558–65.
35. Wysocki AB. Fibronectin in acute and chronic wounds. J ET Nurs 1992;19(5):166–70.
36. Wysocki AB, Staiano-Coico L, Grinnell F. Wound fluid from chronic leg ulcers contains elevated levels of metalloproteinases MMP-2 and MMP-9. J Invest Dermatol 1993; 101(1):64–8.
37. Seah CC, Phillips TJ, Howard CE, et al. Chronic wound fluid suppresses proliferation of dermal fibroblasts through a Ras-mediated signaling pathway. J Invest Dermatol 2005;124(2):466–74.
38. Wysocki AB, Grinnell F. Fibronectin profiles in normal and chronic wound fluid. Lab Invest 1990;63(6):825–31.
39. Yager DR, Zhang LY, Liang HX, et al. Wound fluids from human pressure ulcers contain elevated matrix metalloproteinase levels and activity compared to surgical wound fluids. J Invest Dermatol 1996;107(5):743–8.
40. Philipp K, Riedel F, Germann G, et al. TGF-beta antisense oligonucleotides reduce mRNA expression of matrix metalloproteinases in cultured wound-healing-related cells. Int J Mol Med 2005;15(2):299–303.
41. Philipp K, Riedel F, Sauerbier M, et al. Targeting TGF-beta in human keratinocytes and its potential role in wound healing. Int J Mol Med 2004;14(4):589–93.
42. Riedel K, Riedel F, Goessler UR, et al. TGF-beta antisense therapy increases angiogenic potential in human keratinocytes in vitro. Arch Med Res 2007;38(1):45–51.
43. Sadick H, Herberger A, Riedel K, et al. TGF-beta1 antisense therapy modulates expression of matrix metalloproteinases in keloid-derived fibroblasts. Int J Mol Med 2008;22(1):55–60.
44. Golub LM, McNamara TF, Ryan ME, et al. Adjunctive treatment with subantimicrobial doses of doxycycline: effects on gingival fluid collagenase activity and attachment loss in adult periodontitis. J Clin Periodontol 2001;28(2):146–56.
45. Stechmiller J, Cowan L, Schultz G. The role of doxycycline as a matrix metalloproteinase inhibitor for the treatment of chronic wounds. Biol Res Nurs 2010;11(4):336–44.
46. Robson MC, Mannari RJ, Smith PD, et al. Maintenance of wound bacterial balance. Am J Surg 1999;178(5):399–402.
47. Rodeheaver GT. Pressure ulcer debridement and cleansing: a review of current literature. Ostomy Wound Manage 1999;45(Suppl 1A):80S–5S [quiz: 86S–7S].
48. O'Toole EA. Extracellular matrix and keratinocyte migration. Clin Exp Dermatol 2001;26(6):525–30.
49. Lazarus GS, Cooper DM, Knighton DR, et al. Definitions and guidelines for assessment of wounds and evaluation of healing. Wound Repair Regen 1994;2(3):165–70.
50. Franz MG, Robson MC, Steed DL, et al. Guidelines to aid healing of acute wounds by decreasing impediments of healing. Wound Repair Regen 2008;16(6):723–48.
51. Ueno C, Hunt TK, Hopf HW. Using physiology to improve surgical wound outcomes. Plast Reconstr Surg 2006;117(Suppl 7):59S–71.
52. Kabon B, Rozum R, Marschalek C, et al. Supplemental postoperative oxygen and tissue oxygen tension in morbidly obese patients. Obes Surg 2010;20(7):885–94.
53. O'Mara MS, Hayetian F, Slater H, et al. Results of a protocol of transfusion threshold and surgical technique on transfusion requirements in burn patients. Burns 2005; 31(5):558–61.

54. De Ugarte DA, Roberts RL, Lerdluedeeporn P, et al. Treatment of chronic wounds by local delivery of granulocyte-macrophage colony-stimulating factor in patients with neutrophil dysfunction. Pediatr Surg Int 2002;18(5-6):517–20.

55. Dennis RA, Johnson LE, Roberson PK, et al. Changes in prealbumin, nutrient intake, and systemic inflammation in elderly recuperative care patients. J Am Geriatr Soc 2008;56(7):1270–5.

56. Mast BA, Schultz GS. Interactions of cytokines, growth factors, and proteases in acute and chronic wounds. Wound Repair Regen 1996;4(4):411–20.

57. Bucalo B, Eaglstein WH, Falanga V. Inhibition of cell proliferation by chronic wound fluid. Wound Repair Regen 1993;1(3):181–6.

58. Katz MH, Alvarez AF, Kirsner RS, et al. Human wound fluid from acute wounds stimulates fibroblast and endothelial cell growth. J Am Acad Dermatol 1991;25(6 Pt 1):1054–8.

59. Harris IR, Yee KC, Walters CE, et al. Cytokine and protease levels in healing and non-healing chronic venous leg ulcers. Exp Dermatol 1995;4(6):342–9.

60. Yager DR, Nwomeh BC. The proteolytic environment of chronic wounds. Wound Repair Regen 1999;7(6):433–41.

61. Steed DL, Donohoe D, Webster MW, et al. Effect of extensive debridement and treatment on the healing of diabetic foot ulcers. Diabetic Ulcer Study Group. J Am Coll Surg 1996;183(1):61–4.

62. Harding KG, Moore K, Phillips TJ. Wound chronicity and fibroblast senescence—implications for treatment. Int Wound J 2005;2(4):364–8.

Nutrition and Wound Healing

Jeremy Z. Williams, MD[a], Adrian Barbul, MD[a,b,*]

KEYWORDS

- Nutritional depletion • Wound healing • Immune-related compromise

KEY POINTS

- The relationship between host nutrition and wound healing has been the subject of study and experimentation for centuries, however, wound healing remains enigmatic.
- Nutritional depletion exerts an inhibitory effect, and nutritional supplementation with such positive effectors as arginine can stimulate wound healing.
- Within this paradigm, the physician should be able to recognize patients who may be expected to have wound healing difficulties and offer early intervention to avoid wound failure.

Wound healing and its corresponding intimate relationship to overall nutrition has long been recognized by physicians. The importance of wound healing extends far beyond the scope of medicine, affecting numerous facets of individual and societal life. In the modern era, wound infections and delayed wound healing significantly contribute to the financial burden imposed on health care systems worldwide.

The crucial role of nutrition in cutaneous healing has been recognized since the beginning of medicine as a discipline. Some of the earliest known writings identifying this synergy date to some 2300 years ago, when Hippocrates warned of underestimating the vital role that nutrition played in health and human disease.[1] In the late 1800s, Coleman, Shaffer, and DuBois investigated the metabolic changes occurring in disease.[2] Later, Cuthbertson[3] further defined the biochemical responses to injury by studying patients and animals with long bone fractures. Responses including alterations in physiologic electrolyte levels, increased nitrogen turnover, and stimulation of the overall host metabolism were reported.

In the 1930s, Ravdin, working with other researchers at the University of Pennsylvania, showed the specific relationship between protein malnutrition and the incidence of laparotomy wound dehiscence in dogs.[4–6] Poor nutritional intake or lack of

A version of this article was previously published in *Surgical Clinics* 83:3.
[a] Department of Surgery, Sinai Hospital of Baltimore, 2435 West Belvedere Avenue, Suite 40, Johns Hopkins Medical Institutions, Baltimore, MD 21287, USA; [b] Hackensack University Medical Center, 30 Prospect Avenue- Room 2651, Hackensack, NJ 07601, USA
* Corresponding author. Hackensack University Medical Center, 30 Prospect Avenue- Room 2651, Hackensack, NJ 07601.
E-mail address: abarbul@jhmi.edu

certain essential nutrients significantly alter the body's ability to heal wounds. As interest has swung from understanding the basic physiologic mechanisms of wound healing to attempting to effect some change on the process of wound healing, investigators have explored the ability to modulate the many aspects of wound healing pharmacologically. The dynamic and complicated process of wound healing has proved to be sensitive to external manipulation of metabolic and nutritional factors. The expansion of the ability to deliver select metabolic and nutritional elements has affected greatly the morbidity and mortality of patients sustaining serious injury or wounds.

NUTRITIONAL FACTORS IN WOUND REPAIR
Malnutrition

After injury, many metabolic changes occur that collectively impair wound healing and host defenses. In fact, malnutrition often is deemed to represent only poor or inadequate nutritional intake. Malnutrition encompasses a host of factors from poor nutritional intake to overall metabolic equilibrium. Studies over the past century have shown changes in energy, carbohydrate, protein, fat, vitamin, and mineral metabolism after wounding or injury, each affecting the healing process.[7] Loss of protein from protein-calorie malnutrition leads to decreased wound tensile strength, decreased T-cell function, decreased phagocytic activity, and decreased complement and antibody levels, ultimately diminishing the body's ability to defend the wound against infection. These immune-related compromises of malnutrition correlate clinically with increased wound complication rates and increased wound failure in lower extremity amputations and bypass procedures.[8-10] Malnutrition may preexist wounding or may be encountered secondary to the catabolic imbalance of the patient's overall metabolic state during wound healing. Wounding leads to an increased metabolic rate, increased catecholamine levels, loss of total body water, and increased collagen and other cellular turnover.[11] The host's catabolic response to injury has been shown to be proportional to the severity of the injury.[12,13] The body seems to prioritize healing objectives by metabolic activity. Levenson and others[14-17] showed significantly slower cutaneous wound healing in burned and traumatized animals. Conversely, liver regeneration increased in similarly burned animals. After thermal injury, these disparities in overall anabolic or catabolic state between various organs (ie, liver and skin) suggest that vital organs are preserved at the expense of other organ systems such as the skin. These differences in healing between various organ systems after injury are not well understood, but it is certain that wound healing is impaired as a result of these metabolic changes.

In a society where malnutrition is thought to have been vanquished, a significant proportion of patients do have preexisting malnutrition from decreased nutritional intake. A study of orthopedic patients, including posttrauma patients and patients undergoing total hip replacement, found that 42% of patients were malnourished.[18] A study conducted by Warnold and Lundholm[19] in 1984 evaluated 215 noncancer patients preoperatively and found that 12% showed evidence of malnutrition. Approximately 50% of all medical and surgical patients at an urban hospital in 1974 showed evidence of malnutrition.[20] Although the exact parameters used to define clinical malnutrition may vary, the potential presence of preexisting malnutrition should not be overlooked when assessing a wound or evaluating an unwounded patient about to undergo surgery. Identification of the potential risk imposed by malnutrition is especially important in populations with underlying factors that may impede wound healing further.

An understanding of normal metabolism is helpful when planning an appropriate intervention in patients with malnutrition. One of the most basic elements required for healing is energy, which in the human host is derived from carbohydrates, protein, and fat. Dietary carbohydrates and protein provide approximately 4 kcal/g, and fats provide 9 kcal/g.[21] Reducing caloric intake by 50% in rats decreases collagen synthesis, matrix protein deposition, and granulation tissue formation.[22,23] Although in animal models, severe or prolonged protein-calorie malnutrition is necessary to impair the healing responses, in humans, modest protein-calorie malnutrition impairs fibroplasia.[24] Brief preoperative illness or decreased nutritional intake in the pre-wounding period has been shown to have a significant impact on collagen synthesis. This finding lends support to the concept that preoperative food intake may be more important to the wound healing process than the patient's overall nutritional status.[25] Conversely, brief nutritional intervention by enteral or parenteral routes has been shown to overcome or prevent these impairments in the wound healing process.[26,27]

Although the current literature is laden with studies attempting to delineate the exact role nutrition and supplementation play in the wound healing process, most wounds heal uneventfully. It routinely is observed in the clinical setting that wounds heal despite significant malnutrition. Patients undergoing oncologic operations often present with preoperative weight loss and malnutrition, but these patients generally heal without infection or wound dehiscence. These discrepancies between what has been shown in animal models at the basic science level and what is observed clinically can be reconciled in understanding that the body seems to give a place of preeminence to the healing wound. Albina[28] concluded that the biologic priority of the healing wound accounts for the finding that most wounds heal, even in the face of moderate preoperative and postoperative malnutrition. While establishing this biologic priority of the wound to heal, Albina[28] also noted that severe protein-calorie malnutrition and symptomatic specific nutrient deficiencies can impair wound healing to the extent that they delay the healing process. These findings should not lead clinicians to ignore the need for optimal nutrition. The goal should be to provide every patient with optimal nutrition so that this prioritization of wound healing can occur within an ideal host environment.

Carbohydrates

Carbohydrates, together with fats, are the primary sources of energy in the body and consequently in the wound healing process. The energy requirements for wound healing consist mainly of the energy required to carry out collagen synthesis in the wound. Estimates of caloric requirements for a particular wound can be made knowing that protein synthesis requires 0.9 kcal/g and that a 3 cm^2 ×1 mm thick section of granulation tissue contains 10 mg of collagen. As such, simple wounds have little energy impact on overall metabolism, but large complicated wounds or thermal injuries can divert a disproportionate amount of energy to the healing wound.[29]

Glucose is the major source of fuel used to generate cellular energy in the form of adenosine triphosphate (ATP), which in turn powers the wound healing process. The use of glucose to generate ATP is thought to be relatively inefficient, but the caloric contribution of glucose is essential in preventing the depletion of other amino acid and protein substrates. The liver, triggered by the catecholamine and cortisol surge of wounding, initiates gluconeogenesis using amino acids from degraded muscle protein. Unchecked and in the presence of inadequate carbohydrate and fat stores, this use and depletion of amino acids and protein can lead to the protein-calorie malnutrition previously described. Carbohydrates play an important role in providing the energy essential for optimal healing, but little is known about the function that different sources of carbohydrate play in this process. Gluconeogenesis is an inefficient pathway for glucose production and can result in the production of excess amounts of glucose, which may complicate wound healing, especially in diabetic patients with poor glycemic control.

Diabetic patients often experience significant impairment in the ability to heal wounds and have increased complication rates. The mechanisms at work are multifactorial and poorly understood. The microvascular and atherosclerotic changes induced in diabetics are well known to affect healing. Likewise, diabetes seems to exert an effect on the early inflammatory response and directly inhibits fibroblast and endothelial cell activity. Goodson and Hunt[30] used laboratory animals with streptozotocin-induced diabetes to show a decreased inflammatory response after wounding and diminished fibroblast and endothelial cell proliferation. Delayed epithelialization of open wounds and decreased collagen accumulation deep within the wound have been reported using this diabetic model. Barr and Joyce[31] noted decreased reendothelialization of microarterial anastomoses in streptozotocin diabetic rats and reported that this delay was not alleviated by the adminstration of insulin beginning at the time of surgery and extending into the postoperative period. The relationship of insulin and hyperglycemia to wound healing was clarified on the basis of experiments by Weringer and associates.[32–34] Groups of mice with dermal ear wounds were treated with antiserum to insulin (euglycemic), with 2-deoxyglucose (hyperglycemic), or with food deprivation (hypoglycemic). It was concluded that in addition to hyperglycemia, the lack of insulin itself seems to impair wound healing. Topical application of insulin to infected skin wounds of diabetic mice or systemic administration can improve healing regardless of the route administered.[35] To achieve normal healing, however, the insulin must be given early after wounding.[36] Hyperglycemia also interferes with cellular transport of ascorbic acid into fibroblasts and leukocytes and causes decreased leukocyte chemotaxis.[37]

Mann[38] suggested that a mechanism for this interruption in ascorbic acid transport might be related to the structural similarity between glucose and ascorbic acid, leading to competitive inhibition of ascorbic acid membrane transport. These effects of hyperglycemia in diabetics, specifically as they relate to leukocytes, are thought to help explain the decreased early inflammatory response and impairment of wound healing seen in diabetic patients. It also has been shown that large doses of ascorbic acid administered to streptozotocin-induced diabetic rats can reverse these effects and increase collagen production in the skin. This increase in collagen production after high-dose ascorbic acid administration in diabetic rats is accomplished through reversal of underhydroxylation and degradation and improving intracellular ribosomal collagen production.[39]

The importance of controlling serum glucose levels in diabetics around the time of injury, operation, and wound healing cannot be overemphasized. The alterations in a diabetic's metabolism after injury and after elective surgery can affect wound healing significantly by many of the mechanisms discussed earlier. In addition, diabetic patients are more susceptible to infection because of decreased host resistance. For this reason, it is crucial that physicians recognize and anticipate the needs of diabetic patients early on, before the encumbering effects of diabetes lay hold on the wound healing process.

Fats

In contrast to carbohydrates, the role of fats has not been studied widely. The earliest identification of the importance of fats was a study conducted on animals that were fed a fat-free diet,which became the first clinical description of fat or dietary lipid deficiency.[40,41] Several unsaturated fatty acids must be supplied in the diet. Linoleic acid and arachidonic acid (a product of linoleic acid) are examples of such essential fatty acids. Linolenic acid and arachidonic acid can be synthesized in humans from linoleic acid, but the rates of synthesis are inadequate for basic metabolic needs. As components or precursors of phospholipids and prostaglandins, deficiencies of these lipids cause impairment in wound healing in animals and humans.[42–45] This impairment is due to the role phospholipids play as constituents of the cellular basement membrane and the participation of prostaglandins in cellular metabolism and inflammation.

Demands for essential fatty acids increase after injury.[46,47] Deficiencies of dietary essential fatty acids were not seen frequently clinically until the introduction of prolonged parenteral feedings that did not contain fat. Biochemical changes of essential fatty acid deficiency can manifest within 10 days of eating an entirely fat-free diet.[48] Total parenteral nutrition (TPN) is the most common cause of essential fatty acid deficiency. The administration of TPN results in a rapid onset of essential fatty acid deficiency secondary to the continuous infusion of high concentrations of glucose, which leads to elevated insulin levels, blocking lipolysis and essential fatty acid release.[49]

There also has been research to define further possible benefits of specific lipid types. The ω-3 fatty acids have anti-inflammatory properties by inhibiting eicosanoid production[50–53] and other mediators, such as platelet-activating factor, interleukin-1, and tumor necrosis factor-α.[54,55] Animals consuming diets enriched with ω-3 fatty acids had weaker wounds than controls 30 days after injury. The weaker wounds did not contain less collagen; rather it is thought that the ω-3 supplementation impaired the quality, cross-linking, or spatial orientation of collagen fibrils.

Protein

The importance of protein in wound healing has been recognized and researched since the early 1930s. Under experimental conditions, severe protein deprivation leads to impaired healing. Clinically severe protein malnutrition, known as *kwashiorkor*, is recognized easily. Experimentally, rodents fed either 0% or 4% protein diets showed impaired collagen deposition, decreased skin and fascial wound breaking strength, and increased wound infection rates.[56] Acute protein deprivation in rats has been shown to impair collagen synthesis markedly with a concomitant decrease in procollagen mRNA.[57]

Pure protein deficiencies are seen rarely in the clinical setting. Most patients exhibit combined protein-energy malnutrition or protein-calorie malnutrition. Protein synthesis at the wound site must be increased for collagen deposition and healing to occur. Patients with protein-calorie malnutrition have diminished hydoxyproline accumulation (an index of collagen deposition) in subcutaneously implanted polytetrafluoroethylene catheters compared with normally nourished controls.[58] The administration of individual sulfur-containing amino acids has been shown to abrogate the impaired healing in protein-deficient rats, as evidenced by increased fibroblastic proliferation and collagen accumulation. It is not possible, however, to translate these findings obtained in the context of pure protein deficiency into the setting of protein-calorie malnutrition, which is more clinically prevalent.[59,60]

Amino Acids

Although wound healing can be impaired by deficiencies in a variety of nutrients, there has been a rising interest over the last several decades in the use of individual nutrients to promote wound healing.[29] Often these nutrients are administered in pharmacologic doses that are above the normal daily requirements. In this manner, the role of several single amino acids has been investigated. Two separate studies in the late 1940s and early 1950s showed partial resolution of healing defects in protein-deficient rats with the administration of single sulfur-containing amino acids, such as methionine and cysteine, although the clinical relevance of these findings has never been pursued.[59,60]

Branched-chain amino acids

The branched-chain amino acids valine, leucine, and isoleucine have been used to treat liver disease and have an additional role in retaining nitrogen in sepsis, trauma, and burns.[61-63] Branched-chain amino acids support protein synthesis after injury and decrease muscle proteolysis. Serving as caloric substrates, branched-chain amino acids can be metabolized as an energy source independent of liver function.[64-67] Despite these useful properties, high supplements of branched-chain amino acids have not proved to be of any significant benefit in improving wound healing.[68,69]

Glutamine

Glutamine is the most abundant amino acid in the body, and it accounts for approximately 20% of the total circulating free amino acid pool and 60% of the free intracellular amino acid pool.[70,71] The process of gluconeogenesis involves the shuttling of alanine and glutamine to the liver for conversion to glucose, which is used peripherally as fuel to power certain aspects of wound healing. Glutamine also is an important precursor for the synthesis of nucleotides in cells, including fibroblasts and macrophages.[72,73] Glutamine is as an energy source for lymphocytes and is essential for lymphocyte proliferation.[74,75] Finally, glutamine has a crucial role in stimulating the inflammatory immune response occurring early in wound healing.[76]

Given the abundant roles of glutamine in the numerous cells involved in wound healing, it is not surprising that after injury there is a rapid fall in plasma and muscle glutamine levels,[77,78] which is greater than that of any other amino acid. Although efficacy of supplemental glutamine administration has been shown in some clinical situations,[79] it has not proved to have any noticeable effect on wound healing.[80]

Arginine

In the late 1940s and early 1950s, Rose[81] classified arginine as being one of the two semiessential amino acids in mammalian metabolism. Arginine is a dibasic amino acid that is synthesized endogenously from ornithine through citrulline. It is a normal constituent of numerous body proteins and is associated with a variety of essential reactions of intermediary metabolism. Arginine is absorbed from the intestine by a transport system shared with lysine, ornithine, and cysteine in an energy-dependent and sodium-dependent fashion with substrate specificity. Arginine also shares a common uptake and transport system into fibroblasts and leukocytes with these amino acids.[82]

Arginine is synthesized in adequate quantities to sustain muscle and connective tissue mass but in insufficient quantities for optimal protein biosynthesis and healing. In situations of stress or injury, in which synthesis of arginine is insufficient to meet the demands of increased protein turnover, arginine becomes an indispensable amino acid in the process of wound healing and maintenance of a positive nitrogen balance.[83,84]

The role of arginine in wound healing first was shown in the 1970s, when it was hypothesized that during injury, the amino acid requirements of the adult organism would revert to those of the growing infant. Based on this hypothesis, the effect of arginine deficiency on wound healing in young adult rats was studied. Animals were

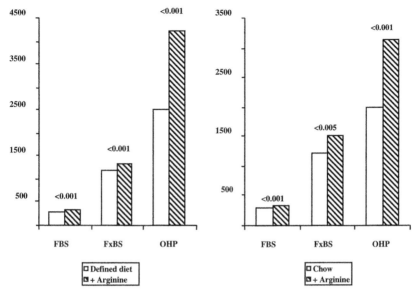

Fig. 1. Effect of supplemental dietary arginine added to an arginine-free (defined) diet or normal laboratory chow (1.8% arginine content) on wound healing in rats. Statistical comparison by Student t-test. FBS, fresh breaking strength of scar, g; FxBS, formalin-fixed breaking strength, g; OHP, hydroxyproline content of subcutaneously implanted polyvinyl alcohol sponges, μg/100 mg sponge dry weight.

fed an arginine-deficient diet for 4 to 6 weeks before wounding. When the animals were subjected to the minor trauma of a dorsal skin incision and closure, they evidenced increased postoperative weight loss, increased mortality to approximately 50%, and a notable decrease in wound breaking strength and wound collagen accumulation compared with animals fed a similarly defined diet containing arginine (**Fig. 1**).[84] Subsequent experiments revealed that chow-fed rats that were not arginine deficient and were fed a diet containing an additional 1% arginine had enhanced wound healing responses as assessed by wound breaking strength and collagen synthesis compared with chow-fed controls (see **Fig. 1**).[84] Similar findings were observed in parenterally fed rats given an amino acid mixture containing high doses (7.5 g/L) of arginine. These animals exhibited increased wound breaking strength, increased collagen accumulation, and enhanced immune function.[85] Likewise, mature or old rats fed diets supplemented with a combination of arginine and glycine have enhanced rates of wound collagen deposition compared with controls.[86]

Several years ago, a micromodel was described that has made possible the study of the human fibroblastic response. In this model, collagen accumulation occurs in a subcutaneously placed 5-cm segment of polytetrafluoroethylene (PTFE) tubing.[87] Two studies were carried out in healthy human volunteers examining the effects of arginine supplementation using this model. In the first study, 36 young, healthy human volunteers (ages 25 to 35) were randomized into one of three groups: (1) 30 g arginine hydrochloride daily supplements (24.8 g free arginine), (2) 30 g arginine aspartate (17 g free arginine), or (3) placebo. The supplements were given for 2 weeks, after which the PTFE catheters were removed and hydroxyproline content (index of reparative collagen synthesis) was evaluated. Arginine supplementation at both doses significantly increased the amount of hydroxyproline and total protein deposition at the

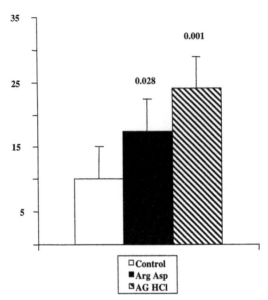

Fig. 2. Effect of 2 weeks of arginine supplementation on hydroxyproline (OHP) accumulation in subcutaneously implanted polytetrafluoroethylene catheters in young human volunteers (mean ± SEM). Groups of 12 volunteers each received a placebo (control), 30 g arginine aspartate (17 g free arginine)/d or 30 g arginine hydrochloride (24.8 g free arginine)/d for 2 weeks.

wound site (**Fig. 2**).[88] The second study evaluated 30 elderly volunteers (age >70) who received 30 g of arginine aspartate (17 g free arginine) or placebo. This study also evaluated the fibroblastic wound response using PTFE catheters and examined epithelialization by creating a split-thickness wound on the upper thigh of each subject. The catheters in this study were analyzed for α-amino nitrogen content (assessment of total protein accumulation), DNA accumulation (index of cellular infiltration), and hydroxyproline content.[90] There was no enhanced DNA present in the wounds of the arginine-supplemented group, suggesting that the effect of arginine is not mediated by an inflammatory mode of action (**Fig. 3**). Arginine supplementation had no effect on the rate of epithelialization of the skin defect, indicating that the predominant effect of arginine is on wound collagen deposition.[89]

Several possible mechanisms have been postulated to explain the positive effect of arginine on wound healing. First, although arginine comprises a small amount of the collagen molecule (<5%), it is possible that supplemental arginine is providing a necessary substrate for collagen synthesis at the wound site. This could be through the direct use of arginine as substrate through the pathway arginine→ornithine→ glutamic semialdehyde→proline. Arginine levels are essentially nondetectable within the wound during the later phases of wound healing when fibroplasia predominates.[90] Although ornithine levels are higher in the wound than in the plasma, further studies by Albina[91] revealed that the rate of conversion of ornithine to proline is quite low, making this mechanism of arginine use unlikely.

Second, it has been observed that the beneficial effects of supplemental arginine on wound healing are similar to the effects of growth hormone, specifically, enhanced wound breaking strength and collagen deposition.[92–94] In a study exploring this

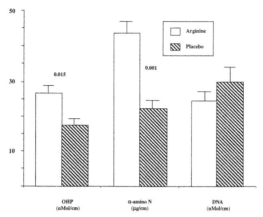

Fig. 3. Effect of arginine on wound healing parameters in healthy elderly human volunteers. Accumulation of hydroxyproline (OHP), total α-amino N, and DNA in subcutaneously implanted polytetrafluoroethylene catheters was measured at the end of 2 weeks (mean $\pm$ SEM). Controls (n = 15) received a placebo syrup; the arginine group (n = 30) received 30 g of arginine aspartate.

observation, hypophysectomized and normal pituitary-bearing animals were divided into two groups—one receiving growth hormone and one receiving placebo treatment—with half of the animals within each group receiving 1% dietary arginine supplementation. After wounding, the intact, arginine-supplemented animals showed increased wound breaking strength and collagen accumulation, whether growth hormone was given or not. In the hypophysectomized animals, arginine had no effect on these wound healing parameters, however, regardless of the administration of growth hormone, suggesting that the effects of arginine on wound healing in rats depend on the presence of an intact hypothalamopituitary axis.[95] In humans, arginine supplementation in doses that are able to increase wound healing also increase plasma insulin-like growth factor, the peripheral mediator of growth hormone.

Third, supplemental arginine has a unique effect on T-cell function. Arginine stimulates T-cell responses and reduces the inhibitory effect of injury and wounding on T-cell function.[85,96–98] T lymphocytes are known to be essential for normal wound healing, as evidenced by decreased wound breaking strength in animals treated with monoclonal antibodies against all T lymphocytes. T lymphocytes are found immunohistochemically throughout the various phases of wound healing in distinctive patterns. Studies have shown that each specific cell type has a modulating role on the phases of cutaneous healing. T lymphocytes interact within the dynamics of each phase of healing to accomplish a specific task, which, when considered collectively, leads to normal repair of the wound.[99] The exact mechanisms are not fully understood, but it is thought that one manner in which arginine may enhance wound healing is by stimulating these host and wound T-cell responses, which in turn would increase fibroplasia.[100–102]

Finally, arginine has been identified as the unique substrate for the generation of the highly reactive radical nitric oxide (NO). Several studies suggest that NO plays a crucial role in wound healing. Inhibitors of NO have been shown to impair significantly healing of cutaneous incisional wounds and colonic anastomosis in rodents.[103,104] In vitro studies have noted increased collagen synthesis in association with exogenous NO administration in cultured dermal fibroblasts.[105] Arginine is catabolized in wounds through two separate pathways: (1) nitric oxide synthases (NOS) and (2) arginase. The liberation of NO from arginine is catabolyzed through the NOS isoenzymes with ultimate production of citrulline. Specifically, it is the inducible isoform iNOS that is activated consistently in response to inflammatory stimuli (eg, wounding). Supranormal collagen deposition has been observed after transfection of iNOS DNA into wounds.[106] Conversely, mice lacking the iNOS gene (iNOS knockout mice) have delayed closure of excisional wounds, an impairment that is remedied by adenoviral transfer of the iNOS gene to the wound bed.[107] The functional loss of the iNOS gene abrogates the beneficial effect of arginine in wound healing, whereas wild-type mice fed arginine-supplemented diets experienced improved incisional wound healing as assessed by breaking strength and collagen deposition. This finding suggests that the iNOS pathway is at least partially responsible for the enhancement of wound healing observed with the administration of arginine.[108]

Vitamins

The vitamins most closely associated with wound healing are vitamin C (ascorbic acid) and vitamin A. Vitamin C deficiency is well known because of its historical significance in relation to scurvy (scorbutus). The earliest accounts of this deficiency were in sailors while at sea and field armies who consumed a diet lacking fresh fruits and vegetables and subsequently developed scurvy. In the late 1800s, Osler[109] categorized and eloquently described the manifestations of this condition, noting that it had virtually disappeared as a clinical entity, owing in large part to the work of Lind. Scurvy has as its central element a failure in collagen synthesis and cross-linking.[110] The symptoms of scurvy reflect this impaired synthesis of collagen and connective tissue and include bleeding into the gingiva, skin, joints, peritoneum, pericardium, and adrenal glands. More generalized symptoms include weakness, fatigue, and depression. During the time that Osler was describing the symptoms of scurvy, the underlying defect in collagen was not understood. Crandon and colleagues[111] first revealed the significance of this "intracellular substance" (collagen) and the temporal aspects of vitamin C deficiency. In 1940, while working as a surgical resident, Crandon consumed a diet lacking vitamin C. After 3 months on this diet, a skin incision healed normally and a biopsy sample at 10 days was normal. At 6 months, a second incision healed poorly, and a 10-day biopsy sample at that time revealed a lack of "intracellular substance." After resuming a diet supplemented with 1 g of ascorbic acid per day, healing improved, and a final biopsy sample showed increased collagen and capillary formation. These early histologic descriptions are consistent with the findings known to be associated with vitamin C deficiency today: minimal collagen, decreased angiogenesis, and significant hemorrhage. Electron microscopy of fibroblasts from scorbutic patients reveals a dilated and disordered rough endoplasmic reticulum with diminished polysome content.[112,113] Ascorbic acid is believed to be a specific cosubstrate for the enzymes 4-hydroxylase and lysyl hydroxylase. From a biochemical standpoint, it is a reducing agent and is required for the conversion of proline and lysine to hydroxyproline and hydroxylysine.[114]

Although the recommended dietary allowance for vitamin C is 60 mg/d, the clinical spectrum of its administration varies widely. In burn victims, the requirement may be 1 to 2 g/d. In human studies, 2 g was required to restore urine and tissue levels to normal after major burn injuries.[115] In animal models, the wounds of burned guinea pigs bore histologic resemblance to those of scorbutic unburned animals. When supplemental vitamin C was given, these changes were prevented. Although the dose needed in different settings may vary, there is no evidence to suggest that massive doses of ascorbic acid are of any substantial benefit to wound healing. There also is no evidence that excess vitamin C is toxic.[116]

Vitamin C deficiency, in addition to impairing wound healing, has been associated with an increased susceptibility to wound infection. If wound infection does occur in the setting of vitamin C deficiency, it is apt to be more severe. These effects are thought to be attributable to the impairment of collagen synthesis interfering with walling-off of bacteria and localizing infection, impairment of neutrophil function, and impairment of complement activity.[29]

McCollum and Davis initially discovered vitamin A in the early 1900s. Subsequent studies in 1941 by Brandaleone and Papper[117] showed the impairment imposed on the wound healing process by vitamin A deficiency. Ehrlich and Hunt[118] described the benefits of supplemental vitamin A on wound healing in nondeficient humans and animals in the 1960s and 1970s. They showed that vitamin A reverses the anti-inflammatory effects of corticosteroids on wound healing. The administration of vitamin A, topically or systemically, also can correct the impaired wound healing of patients on long-term steroid therapy.[119,120] Vitamin A also has been used to restore wound healing impaired by diabetes, tumor formation, cyclophosphamide, or radiation.[121–124]

As alluded to earlier, vitamin A increases the inflammatory response in wounds. This increased response is thought to occur by an enhanced lysosomal membrane lability, increased macrophage influx and activation, and stimulation of collagen synthesis. In vitro studies have shown increased presence of epidermal growth factor receptors and increased collagen synthesis of fibroblast cell cultures in the presence of vitamin A.[125,126] These mechanisms still are not well understood, but it is clear vitamin A plays an important role in wound healing.

Serious injury or stress leads to increased vitamin A requirements. Large doses of corticosteroids also deplete hepatic stores of vitamin A. Decreased serum levels of vitamin A, retinol binding protein, retinyl esters, and β-carotene have been noted after burns, fractures, and elective surgery.[127–129] In the severely injured, doses of vitamin A of 25,000 IU/d (five times the recommended daily dose) have been advocated and used without any significant side effects. Larger doses of vitamin A do not improve further wound healing, and prolonged excessive intake can be toxic.[120]

The fat-soluble vitamin A and the water-soluble vitamin C are the predominant vitamins at work in the wound healing process. The other water-soluble vitamin is vitamin B complex, which seems to play little if any role in wound healing. The B vitamins play an indirect role in wound healing through their influence on host resistance. The remaining fat-soluble vitamins D, E, and K contribute little to wound healing.

Vitamin E maintains and stabilizes cellular membrane integrity, primarily by protection against destruction by oxidation.[130] Vitamin E possesses anti-inflammatory properties, similar to those of steroids, as shown by the reversal of wound healing impairment imposed by vitamin E after administration of vitamin A in the first days after wounding.[131] Vitamin E also has been shown to affect various host immune functions. As an antioxidant, it has been proposed that vitamin E could reduce injury to the wound by excessive free radicals.[120] The liberation of free radicals from inflammatory cascades in necrotic tissue, tissue colonized with microbial flora, ischemic tissue, and chronic wounds can result in depletion of free radical scavengers such as vitamin E.[132,133] This process is believed to be at work in patients with chronic lower extremity wounds. In these patients, it is not known if their relative lack of vitamin E is due to consumption of vitamin E in its antioxidant capacity or overall vitamin E deficiency, either of which could impair healing. In patients with chronic wounds of the lower extremity, some authors suggested that after healing is firmly established, vitamin E may have a role in decreasing excess scar formation, which is known to occur in chronic wounds.[11]

Vitamin K is known as the antihemorrhage vitamin and is required for the carboxylation of glutamate in clotting factors II, VII, IX, and X. Vitamin K contributes little to wound healing, but its absence or deficiency leads to decreased coagulation, which consequently affects the initial phases of healing. Vitamins A and E antagonize the hemostatic properties of vitamin K. Formation of hematomas within the wound can impair healing and predispose to wound infection. This hemostatic capacity of vitamin K influences wound healing.[11]

Micronutrients

Micronutrients are essential components of cellular function and can be divided into organic compounds, such as the vitamins already discussed, and inorganic compounds or trace elements. The term *micronutrients* refers to the extremely small quantities of these compounds found in the body.[130] Although these nutrients comprise only a small portion of the body's overall nutritional needs, their importance is relied on heavily by the cellular machinery that carries out wound healing. It is difficult to associate deficits in specific minerals and trace elements to impairment in wound healing because deficiencies of micronutrients almost always are accompanied by coexisting metabolic or other nutritional disturbances. Most of these minerals and trace elements do not influence wound healing directly; rather they serve as cofactors or part of an enzyme that is essential to healing and homeostasis. Clinicians became more aware of deficiencies of these elements after the introduction of long-term parenteral nutritional solutions, which did not include supplemental minerals and trace elements. As such, it is often easier to prevent these deficiencies than to diagnose them clinically.[29]

Magnesium is a macromineral that is essential for wound repair. Magnesium is a cofactor for many enzymes that are involved in the process of protein synthesis.[11] The primary role of magnesium is to provide structural stability to ATP, which powers many of the processes used in collagen synthesis, making it a factor essential to wound repair.[119,130]

Of the numerous trace elements present in the body, copper, zinc, and iron have the closest relationship to wound healing. Copper is a required cofactor for cytochrome oxidase and the cytosolic antioxidant superoxide dismutase. Lysyl oxidase is a key copper enzyme used in the development of connective tissue, where it catalyzes the cross-linking of collagen and strengthens the collagen framework.[130] Experimentally, impaired healing has been noted secondary to decreased copper stores in patients with Wilson's disease and in animal models after the administration of penicillamine.[134,135]

Zinc is the most well-known element in wound healing and has been used empirically in dermatologic conditions for centuries. Evidence that zinc is essential to wound healing in animals and humans first was described in the rat model in the 1930s and later in humans in the 1950s.[136–139] Zinc is a cofactor for RNA and DNA polymerase and consequently is involved in DNA synthesis, protein synthesis, and cellular proliferation. Zinc deficiency impairs the crucial roles each of these processes play in wound healing. Zinc levels less than 100 μg/100 mL have been associated with impairments in wound healing.[11] In zinc deficiency, fibroblast proliferation and collagen synthesis are decreased, leading to decreased wound strength and delayed epithelialization. These defects are readily reversed with repletion of zinc to normal levels.[29] Immune function is impaired in zinc deficiency. Cellular and humoral elements are impaired, resulting in an increased susceptibility to wound infection and resultant increased possibility of delayed healing. Zinc levels can be depleted in settings of severe stress[140] and in patients receiving long-term steroids. In these settings, it is recommended that patients receive vitamin A and zinc supplements to improve wound healing.[120] The current recommended daily allowance for zinc is 15 mg. No studies have shown improvement in wound healing after the administration of zinc to patients who are not zinc deficient.[141]

Iron is required for the hydroxylation of proline and lysine, and as a result, severe iron deficiency can result in impaired collagen production. As a part of the oxygen transport system, iron can affect wound healing, but this occurs only in settings of severe iron-deficiency anemia. In the clinical setting, iron deficiency is common and can result from blood loss, infectious causes, malnutrition, or an underlying hemato-poietic disorder. In contrast to other deficiencies of trace elements, iron deficiency can be detected and treated easily.[11]

OTHER FACTORS AFFECTING WOUND HEALING
Infection

The complex cascade of events discussed earlier, which comprise the body's response to tissue injury with the purpose of restoring cutaneous integrity, occurs in the presence of various environmental factors. Any of these factors can impair the wound healing process if not effectively managed or prevented.

Sepsis, whether present as local bacterial colonization of the wound site or as a systemic inflammatory response, is one of the most formidable "environmental" obstacles to successful wound healing. Experimentally the crucial inoculum of microorganisms that significantly inhibits healing has been determined to be 10^5 colony-forming units/cm^2 wound surface or gram of tissue.[142,143] In addition to appropriate antibiotic therapy, an intact, functioning immune system is vital to preventing and clearing wound infection. The immune system is tied to overall host nutrition and specific nutritional entities, such as arginine and its related metabolic pathways. In critically ill patients, it is crucial that nutritional status be optimized to provide increased substrate availability to meet the demands of tissue repair and immune function and to prevent wounds from succumbing to infection and delayed healing.[144]

Evaluation of Overall Nutritional State

Clinicians must be aware of nutritional disturbances in wounded patients before these nutritional deficits can be corrected. The severity of the deficit must be assessed, and the caloric requirements for healing to ensue should be estimated. Kinney[145] outlined the metabolic adjustments experienced after injury as follows: (1) uncomplicated intra-abdominal surgery increases metabolic rate approximately 10%; (2) uncompli-cated injuries, such as femoral fracture, increase metabolism about 20%; (3) peritonitis increases metabolism 20% to 40%; (4) third-degree burns increase metabolism 50% to 100%; and (5) fever alone increases metabolism 10% for each 1°C. Historically the *sine qua non* of linear nutritional status over time has been serial weight measurements. This commonly used marker for malnutrition can be mislead-ing, however, if the presence of abnormal amounts of body water is not taken into account. Total body water increases at approximately the same rate body protein decreases.[146] Body water also can influence the anthropometric measurements used to estimate body fat from skin-fold thickness and predetermined nomograms.

Other markers predictive of nutritional state include serum albumin and transferrin levels, total lymphocyte count, anergy-delayed hypersensitivity, urinary nitrogen, and respiratory minute volume. One of the least expensive and practical ways to estimate simple caloric requirements of seriously ill patients is respiratory minute volume. In the absence metabolic acidosis or alkalosis, with normal breathing the respiratory minute volume gives a close correlation to the patient's metabolic rate. This information can be used to guide nutritional care. Serum albumin levels and total lymphocyte count also are useful nutritional prognosticators. In a study of nutritional status as a predictor of wound healing after amputation, normal albumin and total lymphocyte levels correlated with increased rates of healing.[147] These values also can be misinterpreted, however, if factors such as liver dysfunction, sepsis, or infection are present and not taken into account. Depressed hypersensitivity reactions to intradermally injected antigens also has been established as an indicator of nutritional status.[148]

Feeding

Wound healing has been described repeatedly in this article as a complex series of cellular and biochemical events that are interdependent on the availability of energy. The substrate for the production of this wound healing energy is protein, carbohydrate, fat, amino acids, and micronutrients, which have been described previously. Specifically, it has been recommended that the calorie-to-nitrogen ratio be 120 to 150:1 during the early weeks of wound healing after severe injury, then raised to 200 to 225:1 as the body shifts to a period of positive nitrogen balance.[149]

Patients who are malnourished before wounding have increased rates of wound infection and delayed wound healing. There seems to be ample evidence that nutritional repletion before planned elective operations in malnourished patients significantly reduces these complications. The exact route of administration, whether it is enteral or parenteral, may be important, but the existing data are conflicting.

TPN has been shown to reduce postoperative complications when administered to severely malnourished patients for at least 7 days preoperatively.[150,151] TPN has many associated risks, however, not the least of which is infection. Total enteral nutrition (TEN) also has associated risks, but there is growing experimental evidence that TEN is superior to TPN as a feeding modality. Studies evaluating the route of nutrition and wound healing in rats showed that TEN particularly influences the early stages of wound healing. In these studies, TEN significantly increased collagen deposition and wound breaking strength compared with TPN 5 days after wounding (**Fig. 4**). This beneficial influence seems to disappear during the period of maximal fibroplasias, which occurs 5 to 10 days after injury. TEN seems to maintain local and systemic immune responses; preserves gut integrity, decreasing bacterial translocation; and improves protein metabolism and survival.[152–155] As already alluded to, TEN seems to exert a greater influence over the early cellular, inflammatory phase of wound healing than does TPN. This cellular phase is exquisitely sensitive to nutrient availability. The influence TEN has on systemic immune function contributes to the function and number of inflammatory cells present during early healing, ultimately affecting wound repair.[156]

The exact feeding regimen should be tailored to each individual patient. In patients who are malnourished, preoperative repletion should be accomplished by the route that exposes the patient to the least risk, and if possible, elective operations should be delayed until the patient is satisfactorily supplemented. In patients who are not likely to take nutrition orally, TPN should be initiated early. The nutritional supplement should be as specific as possible to the patient's perceived nutritional deficiency, and substrates that are turned over rapidly should be included. The amino acid arginine as previously discussed is turned over rapidly in wound healing. Of greatest importance is that nutritional deficiencies be recognized early and that repletion be initiated early

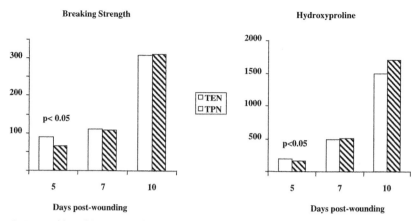

Fig. 4. Wound breaking strength (g, mean ± SEM) and hydroxyproline content (µg/100 mg sponge, mean ± SEM) of the sponge granulomas in enterally (total enteral nutrition [TEN]) and parenterally (total parenteral nutrition [TPN]) ▨ fed animals.

because even brief periods of malnutrition can have significant negative effects on wound healing.

SUMMARY

The relationship between host nutrition and wound healing has been the subject of study and experimentation for centuries. Despite the many years of study and a substantial knowledge base of the specific processes and factors involved, wound healing remains enigmatic. There is still much to learn about the wound-specific nutritional interventions that are available to improve wound healing. Nutrition profoundly influences the process of wound healing. Nutritional depletion exerts an inhibitory effect, and nutritional supplementation with such positive effectors as arginine can stimulate wound healing. Within this paradigm, the physician should be able to recognize patients who may be expected to have wound healing difficulties and offer early intervention to avoid wound failure.

REFERENCES

1. Hippocrates. The genuine works of Hipocrates (translated from the Greek by Francis Adams). Baltimore: Williams & Wilkins; 1939.
2. DuBois EF. Metabolism in fever and in certain infections. In: Barker LF, editor. Endocrinology and metabolism, vol IV, D. New York: Appleton; 1922. p. 95–151.
3. Cuthbertson DP. The biochemical response to injury. Springfield (IL): Charles C Thomas; 1960.
4. Thompson WD, Ravdin IS, Frank IL. The effect of hypoproteinemia on wound disruption. Arch Surg 1938;36:500.
5. Thompson WD, Ravdin IS, Rhoads JE, et al. The use of lyophile plasma incorrection of hypoproteinemia and prevention of wound disruption. Arch Surg 1938;36:509.
6. Rhoads JE, Fliegelman MT, Panzer LM. The mechanism of delayed wound healing in the presence of hypoproteinemia. JAMA 1942;118:21.
7. Levenson SM, Demetriou AA. Metabolic factors. In: Wound healing biochemical and clinical aspects. Philadelphia: WB Saunders; 1992. p. 248–73.

8. Kay SP, Moreland JR, Schmitler E. Nutritional status and wound healing in lower extremity amputations. Clin Orthop 1987;217:253.

9. Dickhaut SC, DeLee JC, Page CP. Nutritional status: importance in predicting wound healing after amputation. J Bone Joint Surg Am 1984;66:71.

10. Casey J, Flinn WR, Yao JS, et al. Correlation of immune and nutritional status with wound complications in patients undergoing vascular operations. Surgery 1983;93:822.

11. Fischer JE. Nutrition and metabolism in the surgical patient. Boston: Little, Brown; 1996.

12. Cuthbertson DP. Nutrition in relation to trauma and surgery. Prog Nutr Sci 1975;1:263.

13. Bessey PQ. Metabolic response to critical illness. In: Wilmore DW, Cheung LY, Harken AH, editors. Scientific American Surgery: Care of the surgical patient. New York: WebMD Corporation; 1999. p. 1–26.

14. Levenson SM, Pirani CL, Braasch JW, et al. The effect of thermal burns on wound healing. Surg Gynecol Obstet 1954;99:74.

15. Levenson SM, Upjohn HL, Preston JA. Effect of thermal burns on wound healing. Ann Surg 1957;146:357.

16. Crowley LV, Seifter E, Kriss P, et al. Effects of environmental temperature and femoral fracture on wound healing in rats. J Trauma 1977;17:436.

17. Levenson SM, Crowley LV, Oates JF, et al. Effect of severe burn on liver regeneration. Surg Forum 1958;9:493.

18. Jensen JE, Jensen TG, Smith TK, et al. Nutrition in orthopaedic surgery. J Bone Joint Surg AM 1982;64:1263.

19. Warnold I, Lundholm K. Clinical significance of preoperative nutritional status in 215 noncancer patients. Ann Surg 1984;199:299.

20. Daley BJ, Bistrian BR. Nutritional assessment. In: Zaloga GP, editor. Nutrition in critical care. St. Louis Mosby 1994. p. 9–33.

21. Schwartz SI. Principles of surgery. New York: McGraw-Hill; 1994.

22. Yue DK, McLennan S, Marsh M, et al. Abnormalities of granulation tissue and collagen formation in experimental diabetes, uremia and malnutrition. Diabet Med 1986;3:221.

23. Spanheimer RG, Peterkovsky B. A specific decrease in collagen synthesis in acutely fasted, vitamin C–supplemented, guinea pigs. J Parenter Enteral Nutr 1986;10:550.

24. Goodson WH 3rd, Lopez-Sarmiento A, Jensen JA, et al. The influences of a brief preoperative illness on postoperative healing. Ann Surg 1987;205:250.

25. Windsor JA, Knoght GS, Hill GL. Wound healing response in surgical patients: recent food intake is more important than nutritional status. Br J Surg 1988;75:135.

26. Haydock DA, Hill GL. Improved wound healing response in surgical patients receiving intravenous nutrition. Br J Surg 1987;74:320.

27. Schroeder D, Gillanders L, Mahr R, et al. Effects of immediate postoperative nutrition in body composition, muscle function and wound healing. J Parenter Enteral Nutr 1991;15:376.

28. Albina JE. Nutrition and wound healing. J Parenter Enteral Nutr 1994;18:367.

29. Barbul A, Purtill WA. Nutrition in wound healing. Clin Dermatol 1994;12:133.

30. Goodson WH III, Hunt TK. Wound collagen accumulation in obese hyperglycemic mice. Diabetes 1986;35:491.

31. Barr LC, Joyce AD. Microvascular anastamoses in diabetes: an experimental study. Br J Plast Surg 1989;42:50.

32. Weringer EJ, Kelso JM, Tamai IY, et al. Effects of insulin in wound healing in diabetic mice. Acta Endocrinol 1982;99:101.

33. Weringer EJ, Arquilla ER. Wound healing in normal and diabetic Chinese hamsters. Diabetologia 1981;4:394.
34. Weringer EJ, Kelso JM, Tamai IY, et al. The effect of antisera to insulin, 2-deoxyglucose-induced hyperglycemia and starvation on wound healing in normal mice. Diabetes 1981;30:407.
35. Hanam SR, Singleton CE, Rudek W. The effect of topical insulin on infected cutaneous ulcerations in diabetic and nondiabetic mice. J Foot Surg 1983;22:298.
36. Goodson WH, Hunt TK. Studies of wound healing in experimental diabetes mellitus. J Surg Res 1977;22:221.
37. Mann GV. The impairment of transport of amino acid by monosaccharides [abstract]. Fed Proc 1974;33:251.
38. Mann GV. The membrane transport of ascorbic acid. Ann N Y Acad Sci 1974;258:243.
39. Schneir M, Rettura G, et al. Dietary ascorbic acid increases collagen production in skin of stretozotocin induced diabetic rats by normalizing ribosomal efficiency. Ann N Y Acad Sci 1987;194:42.
40. Burr GO, Burr MM. A new deficiency disease produced by the rigid exclusion of fat from the diet. J Biol Chem 1929;82:345.
41. Burr GO, Burr MM. On the nature and role of the fatty acids essential in nutrition. J Biol Chem 1930;86:587.
42. Hulsey TK, O'Neill JA, Neblett WR, et al. Experimental wound healing in essential fatty acid deficiency. J Pediatr Surg 1980;15:505.
43. Caffrey BB, Jonnson JT Jr. Role of essential fatty acids in wound healing in rats. Prog Lipid Res 1981;20:641.
44. Caldwell MD, Jonsson HT, Othersen HB Jr. Essential fatty acid deficiency in an infant receiving prolonged parenteral alimentation. J Pediatr 1972;81:894.
45. Nordenstrom J, Carpentier YA, Askanazi J, et al. Essential fatty acid deficiency and apparent wound healing in an infant with gastroschisis. Am Surg 1983;197:725.
46. Wolfram G, Eckart J, Walther B, et al. Free fatty acid mobilization and oxidation during total parenteral nutrition in trauma and infection. Ann Surg 1983;198:275.
47. Wolfram G, Eckart J, Walther B, et al. Factors influencing essential fatty acid requirements in total parenteral nutrition. J Parenter Enteral Nutr 1978;2:634.
48. Wene JD, Connor WE, DenBesten L. The development of essential fatty acid deficiency in men fed fat free diets intravenously and orally. J Clin Invest 1975;56:127.
49. Greig PD, Baker JP, Jeejeebhoy KN. Metabolic effects of total parenteral nutrition. Annu Rev Nutr 1982;2:179.
50. Albina JE, Gladden P, Walsh WR. Detrimental effects of omega-3 fatty acid-enriched diet on wound healing. J Parenter Enteral Nutr 1993;17:519.
51. Simopoulos AL. Omega-3 fatty acids in health and disease and in growth and development. Am J Clin Nutr 1993;54:438.
52. Prickett JD, Robinson DR, Steinberg AD. Effects of dietary enrichment with eicosapentanoic acid upon autoimmune nephritis in female NZBxNZW/F1 mice. Arthritis Rheum 1983;26:133.
53. Kremer JM, Jubiz W, Michalek A, et al. Fish oil fatty acid supplementation in active rheumatoid arthritis: a double-blind, controlled, crossover study. Ann Intern Med 1987;106:497.
54. Sperling RI, Robin JL, Kylander KA, et al. The effects of N-3 polyunsaturated fatty acids on the generation of platelet-activating factor by human monocytes. J Immunol 1987;139:4186.

55. Endres S, Ghorbani R, Kelly VE, et al. The effect of dietary supplementation with N-3 polyunsaturated fatty acids on the synthesis of interleukin-1 and tumor necrosis factor by mononuclear cells. N Engl J Med 1989;320:265.

56. Irvin TT. Effects of malnutrition and hyperalimentation on wound healing. Surg Gynecol Obstet 1978;146:33.

57. Spanheimer RG, Peterkovsky B. A specific decrease in collagen synthesis in acutely fasted, vitamin C–supplemented, guinea pigs. J Biol Chem 1985;260:3955.

58. Haydock GA, Hill GL. Impaired wound healing in surgical patients with varying degrees of malnutrition. J Parenter Enteral Nutr 1986;10:550.

59. Williamson MB, Fromm HJ. The incorporation of sulfur amino acids into protein of regenerating wound tissue. J Biol Chem 1955;212:705.

60. Localio SA, Morgan ME, Hintown R. The biological chemistry of wound healing: the effect of di-methionine on healing of wounds in protein depleted animals. Surg Gynecol Obstet 1948;86:582.

61. Cerra FB, Upson D, Angelico R, et al. Branched chains support postoperative protein synthesis. Surgery 1982;92:192.

62. Cerra FB, Shronts EP, Konstantinides NN, et al. Enteral feeding in sepsis: a prospective, randomized double blind trial. Surgery 1985;98:632.

63. Sax HC, Talamini MA, Fischer JE. Clinical use of branched chain amino acids in liver disease, trauma, sepsis and burns. Arch Surg 1986;121:358.

64. Cerra FB, Siegel JH, Coleman B, et al. Septic autocannibalism: a failure of exogenous nutritional support. Ann Surg 1980;192:570.

65. Hedden MP, Buse MG. General stimulation of muscle protein synthesis by branched chain amino acids in vitro. Proc Soc Exp Biol Med 1979;160:410.

66. Buse MG, Reid SS. Leucine, a possible regulator of protein turnover in muscles. J Clin Invest 1975;56:1250.

67. Freund HR, Lapidot A, Fischer JE. The use of branched chain amino acids in the injured-septic patient. In: Walser M, Williamson JR, editors. Metabolism and clinical implications of branch chain amino and ketoacids. New York: Elsevier; 1981. p. 527–32.

68. McCauley R, Platell C, Hall J, et al. Influence of branched chain amino acid solutions on wound healing. Aust N Z J Surg 1990;60:471.

69. Dudrick SJ, Matheny RG, et al. Effect of enriched branched chain amino acid solutions in traumatized rats [abstract]. J Parenter Enteral Nutr 1984;8:86.

70. Demling RH, Desanti L. Involuntary weight loss and the nonhealing wound: the role of anabolic agents. Adv Wound Care 1999;12(Suppl):1.

71. Bergstrom J, Furst P, Noree LO, et al. Intracellular free amino acid concentration in human muscle tissue. J Appl Physiol 1974;36:693.

72. Zetterberg A, Engstrom W. Glutamine and the regulation of DNA replication and cell multiplication in fibroblasts. J Cell Physiol 1981;108:365.

73. Zielke HR, Ozand PT, Tildon JT, et al. Growth of human diploid fibroblasts in the absence of glucose utilization. Proc Natl Acad Sci U S A 1976;73:4110.

74. Ardawi MSM, Newsholme P. Glutamine metabolism in lymphocytes of the rat. Biochem 1983;212:835–42.

75. Newsholme EA, Newsholme P. A role for muscle in the immune system and its importance in surgery, trauma, sepsis and burns. Nutrition 1988;4:261.

76. Demling RH. Desanti L. Involuntary weight loss and the nonhealing wound: the role of anabolic agents. Adv Wound Care 1999;12(Suppl):1.

77. Askanazi J, Carpentier YA, Michelsen CB, et al. Muscle and plasma amino acids following injury: influence of intercurrent infection. Ann Surg 1980;192:78.

78. Roth E, Funovics J. Metabolic disorders in sever abdominal sepsis: glutamine deficiency in skeletal muscle. Clin Nutr 1982;1:25.
79. Ziegler TR, Young LS, Benfell K, et al. Clinical and metabolic efficacy of glutamine-supplemented parenteral nutrition after bone marrow transplant. A randomized, double-blind, controlled study. Ann Intern Med 1992;116:821.
80. McCauly R, Platell C, Hall J, et al. Effects of glutamine on colonic strength anastamosis in the rat. J Parenter Enteral Nutr 1991;15:437.
81. Rose WC. The nutritive significance of the amino acids and certain related compounds. Science 1937;86:298.
82. Barbul A. Biochemistry, physiology and therapeutic implications. J Parenter Enteral Nutr 1986;10:227.
83. Rose WC. Amino acid requirements of man. Fed Proc 1949;8:546.
84. Seifter E, Rettura G, Barbul A, et al. Arginine: an essential amino acid for injured rats. Surgery 1978;84:224.
85. Barbul A, Fishel RS, Shimazu S, et al. Intravenous hyperalimentation with high arginine levels improves wound healing and immune function. J Surg Res 1985;38:328.
86. Chyun J, Griminger P. Improvement of nitrogen retention by arginine and glycine supplementation and its relation to collagen synthesis. J Nutr 1984;114:1697.
87. Goodson WH, Hunt TK. Development of a new miniature method for the study of wound healing in human subjects. J Surg Res 1982;33:394.
88. Barbul A, Lazarou SA, Efron DT, et al. Arginine enhances wound healing and lymphocyte immune response in humans. Surgery 1991;108:331.
89. Kirk SJ, Hurston M, Regan MC, et al. Arginine stimulates wound healing and immune function in elderly human beings. Surgery 1993;114:155.
90. Albina JE, Mills CD, Barbul A, et al. Arginine metabolism in wounds. Am J Phys 1988;254:E459.
91. Albina JE, Mastrofrancesco B. Role of ornithine as proline precursor in healing wounds. J Surg Res 1993;55:97.
92. Kowalewski K, Young S. Effect of growth hormone and an anabolic steroid on hydroxyproline in healing dermal wounds in rats. Acta Endocrinol 1968;59:53.
93. Jorgensen PH, Andreassen TT. Influence of biosynthetic human growth hormone on biochemical properties of rat skin incisional wounds. Acta Chir Scand 1988;154:623.
94. Herndon DN, Barrow RE, Kunkel KR, et al. Effects of recombinant human growth hormone on donor site-healing in severely burned children. Ann Surg 1990;212:424.
95. Barbul A, Rettura G, Levenson SM, et al. Wound healing and thymotropic effects of arginine: a pituitary mechanism of action. Am J Clin Nutr 1983;37:786.
96. Barbul A, Wasserkrug HL, Seifter E, et al. Immunostimulatory effects of arginine in normal and injured rats. J Surg Res 1980;29:228.
97. Barbul A, Wassekrug HL, Sisto DA, et al. Thymic stimulatory actions of arginine. J Parenter Enteral Nutr 1980;4:446.
98. Barbul A, Wasserkrug HL, Yoshimura N, et al. High arginine levels in intravenous hyperalimentation abrogate post-traumatic immune suppression. J Surg Res 1984;36:620.
99. Agaiby AD, Dyson M. Immuno-inflammatory cell dynamics during cutaneous wound healing. J Anat 1999;195:531.
100. Fishel RS, Barbul A, Beschorner WE, et al. Lymphocyte participation in wound healing: morphologic assessment using monoclonal antibodies. Ann Surg 1987;206:25.

101. Peterson JM, Barbul A, Breslin RJ, et al. Significance of T lymphocytes in wound healing. Surgery 1987;102:300.
102. Barbul A. Role of T cell-dependent immune system in wound healing. In: Growth factors and other aspects of wound healing: biologic and clinical implications. New York: Alan R. Liss; 1988. p. 161–75.
103. Schaffer MR, Tantry U, Thornton FJ, et al. Inhibition of nitric oxide synthesis in wounds: pharmacology and effect on accumulation of collagen in wounds in mice. Eur J Surg 1999;165:262.
104. Efron DT, Thornton FJ, Steulten C, et al. Expression and function of inducible nitric oxide synthase during rat colon anastomotic healing. J Gastrointest Surg 1999;3: 592.
105. Schaffer MR, Efron PA, Thornton FJ, et al. Nitric oxide, an autocrine regulator of wound fibroblast synthetic function. J Immunol 1997;158:2375.
106. Thornton FJ, Schaffer MR, Witte MB, et al. Enhanced collagen accumulation following direct transfection of the inducible nitric oxide synthase gene in cutaneous wounds. Biochem Biophys Res Commun 1998;246:654.
107. Yamasaki K, Edington HD, McClosky C, et al. Reversal of impaired wounds repair in iNOS deficient mice by topical adenoviral-mediated iNOS gene transfer. J Clin Invest 1998;101:967.
108. Shi HP, Efron DT, Most D, et al. Supplemental dietary arginine enhances wound healing in normal but not inducible nitric oxide synthase knockout mice. Surgery 2000;128:374.
109. Osler W. The principles and practice of medicine. D. Appleton & Company: New York; 1892.
110. Englard S, Seifter E. The biochemical functions of ascorbic acid. Annu Rev Nutr 1986;6:365.
111. Crandon JH, Lund CC, Dill DB, et al. Experimental human scurvy. N Engl J Med 1940;223:353.
112. Lanman TH, Ingalls TH. Vitamin C deficiency and wound healing (experimental and clinical study). Ann Surg 1937;105:516.
113. Bourne GH. Effect of vitamin C deficiency on experimental wounds: tensile strength and histology. Lancet 1944;1:688.
114. Kivirikko KI, Helaakoski T, Tasanen K, et al. Molecular biology of prolyl 4-hydroxy-lase. Ann N Y Acad Sci 1990;580:132.
115. Lund CC, Levenson SM, Green RW, et al. Ascorbic acid, thiamine riboflavin and nicotinic acid in relation to acute burns in man. Arch Surg 1947;55:557.
116. Rivers JM. Safety of high level vitamin C injection. Ann N Y Acad Sci 1987;498:445.
117. Brandaleone H, Papper E. The effect of the local and oral administration of cod liver oil on the rate of wound healing in vitamin A deficient and normal animals. Ann Surg 1941;114:791.
118. Ehrlich HP, Hunt TK. Effects of cortisone and vitamin A on wound healing. Ann Surg 1968;167:324.
119. Levenson SM, Seifter E, VanWinkle W. Nutrition. In: Hunt TK, Dunphy JE, editors. Fundamentals of wound management in surgery. New York: Appleton-Century-Crofts; 1979. p. 286–363.
120. Goodson WH, III, Hunt TK. Wound healing and nutrition. In: Kinney JM, Jeejeebhoy KN, Hill GL, editors. Nutrition and metabolism in patient care. Philadelphia: WB Saunders; 1988. p. 635–42.
121. Seifter E, Rettura G, Padawer J, et al. Impaired wound healing in streptozotocin diabetes: prevention by supplemental vitamin A. Ann Surg 1981;194:42.

122. Weinzweig J, Levenson SM, Rettura G, et al. Supplemental vitamin A prevents the tumor induced defect in wound healing. Ann Surg 1990;211:269.
123. Stratford F, Seifter E. Impaired wound healing by cyclophosphamide: alleviation by supplemental vitamin A. Surg Forum 1980;31:224.
124. Levenson SM, Gruber CA, Rettura G, et al. Supplemental vitamin A prevents the acute radiation-induced defect in wound healing. Ann Surg 1984;200:494.
125. Demetriou AA, Levenson SM, Rettura G, et al. Vitamin A and retinoic acid: induced fibroblast differentiation in vitro. Surgery 1985;98:931.
126. Jetten AM. Modulation of cell growth by retinoids and their possible mechanisms of action. Fed Proc 1984;43:134.
127. Moody BJ. Changes in the serum concentrations of thyroxine-binding prealbumin and retinol binding protein following burn injury. Clin Chim Act 1982;118:87.
128. Rai K, Coutemanche AJ. Vitamin A assay in burned patients. J Trauma 1975;15:419.
129. Ramsden DB, Prince HP, Burr WA, et al. The interrelationship of thyroid hormones, vitamin A and the binding proteins following stress. Clin Endocrinol 1978;8:109.
130. Demling RH, DeBiasse M. Micronutrients in critical illness. Crit Care Clin 1995;11: 651.
131. Hunt TK. Vitamin A and wound healing. J Am Acad Dermatol 1986;15:817.
132. Baxter CR. Immunologic reactions in chronic wounds. Am J Surg 1994;167:12.
133. Shukla A, Rasik AM, Patnaik GK. Depletion of reduced glutathione, ascorbic acid, and vitamin E and antioxidant defense enzymes in a healing cutaneous wound. Free Radic Res 1997;26:93.
134. Nimni ME. Mechanism of collagen crosslinking by penicillamine. Proc R Soc Med 1977;70:65.
135. Geever EF, Youssef SA, Seifter E, et al. Penicillamine and wound healing in young guinea pigs. J Surg Res 1967;6:160.
136. Todd WR, Elvehjem CA, Hart EB. Zinc in nutrition of the rat. Am J Physiol 1934;107: 146.
137. Vallee BL. Metabolic role of zinc: report of Council of Foods and Nutrition. JAMA 1956;162:1053.
138. Ramsden DB, Prince HP, Burr WA, et al. The interrelationship of thyroid hormones, vitamin A and their binding proteins following stress. Clin Endocrinol 1978;8:109.
139. Prasad AS, Miale A. Biochemical studies on dwarfism, hypogonadism and anemia. Arch Intern Med 1963;111:407.
140. Prasad AS. Acquired zinc deficiency and immune dysfunction in sickle cell anemia. In: Cunningham-Rundles S, editor. Nutrient modulation of the immune response. New York: Marcel Dekker; 1993. p. 393–410.
141. Hallbrook T, Lanner E. Serum zinc and healing of leg ulcers. Lancet 1972;2:780.
142. Raahave D, Friis-Moller A, Bjerre-Jepsen K, et al. The infective dose of aerobic and anaerobic bacteria in postoperative wound sepsis. Arch Surg 1986;121:924.
143. Robson MC, Shaw RC, Heggers JP. The reclosure of postoperative incisional abcesses based on bacterial quantification of the wound. Ann Surg 1970;171:279.
144. Thornton FJ, Schaffer MR, Barbul A. Wound healing in sepsis and trauma. Shock 1997;8:391.
145. Kinney JM. Energy requirements of the surgical patient. In: Ballinger WF, Collins JA, Druker WR, editors. Manual of surgical nutrition. Philadelphia: WB Saunders; 1975. p. 223–35.
146. Streats SJ, Hill GL. Nutritional support in the management of critically ill patients in surgical intensive care. World J Surg 1987;11:194.
147. Dickhaut SC, DeLee JC, Page CP. Nutritional status: importance in predicting wound healing after amputation. J Bone Joint Surg Am 1984;66:71.

148. Christou N. Perioperative nutritional support: immunologic defects. J Parenter Enteral Nutr 1990;14:186S.
149. Levenson SM, Seifter E, Walton VW. Fundamentals of wound management in surgery. South Plainfield (NJ): Chirurgecom; 1977.
150. Mullen JL, Buzby GP, Matthews DC, et al. Reduction of operative morbidity and mortality by combined preoperative and postoperative nutritional support. Ann Surg 1980;192:604.
151. Williams RH, Heatley RV, Lewis MH. Proceedings: a randomized control trial of preoperative intravenous nutrition in patients with stomach cancer. Br J Surg 1976;6:667.
152. Zaloga GP, Knowles R, Black KW, et al. TPN increases mortality after hemorrhage. Crit Care Med 1991;19:54.
153. Kudsk KA, Stone JM, Carpenter G, et al. Enteral and parenteral nutrition influences mortality after hemoglobin-*E. coli* peritonitis in normal rats. J Trauma 1983;23:605.
154. Delany HM, John J, Teh EL, et al. Contrasting effects of identical nutrients given parenterally or enterally after 70% hepatectomy. Am J Surg 1994;167:135.
155. Lin MT, Saito H, Fukushima R, et al. Route of nutritional supple influences local, systemic and remote organ responses to intraperitoneal bacterial challenge. Ann Surg 1996;223:84.
156. Kiyama T, Witte MB, Thornton FJ, et al. The route of nutrition support affects the early phase of wound healing. J Parenter Enteral Nutr 1998;22:276.

The Impact of Psychological Stress on Wound Healing:
Methods and Mechanisms

Jean-Philippe Gouin, PhD[a],*, Janice K. Kiecolt-Glaser, PhD[b,c]

KEYWORDS

- Wound healing • Stress • Cytokine • Cortisol • Psychoneuroimmunology • Oxytocin

KEY POINTS

- The goal of this review is to present clinical and experimental models of the impact of stress on wound repair.
- Converging and replicated evidence from experimental and clinical models of wound healing indicates that psychological stress leads to clinically relevant delays in wound healing.
- Translational work should focus on identifying conditions in which behavioral and pharmacologic treatments are the most effective and on developing new treatments able to attenuate stress-induced delays in wound healing.

Wound healing is a critical process involved in the recovery from injury and surgical procedures. Poor healing increases the risk for wound infections or complications, lengthens hospital stays, magnifies patient discomfort, and slows return to activities of daily living. Converging evidence from different research paradigms suggests that psychological stress and other behavioral factors can affect wound healing. A meta-analytical study using diverse wound-healing models and outcomes found that across studies there was an average correlation of −0.42 between psychological stress and wound healing.[1] This result suggests that the relationship between stress and wound repair is not only statistically significant but also clinically relevant. This

A version of this article was previously published in *Immunology and Allergy Clinics* 31:1.
Work on this article was supported by a doctoral research training award from the Fonds de la Recherche en Santé du Québec and NIH grants AG029562, CA126857, CA131029, AT003912, Ohio State Comprehensive Cancer Center Core Grant CA16058, and NCRR Grant UL1RR025755.
[a] Department of Psychology, Concordia University, 7141 Sherbrooke Street West, PY 170-14, Montreal, QC H4B 1R6, Canada; [b] Institute for Behavioral Medicine Research, The Ohio State University College of Medicine, 460 Medical Center Drive, Room 139, Columbus, OH 43210-1228, USA; [c] Department of Psychiatry, The Ohio State University College of Medicine, 1670 Upham Drive, Columbus, OH 43210, USA
* Corresponding author.
E-mail address: jp.gouin@concordia.ca

Crit Care Nurs Clin N Am 24 (2012) 201–213
doi:10.1016/j.ccell.2012.03.006
0899-5885/12/$ – see front matter © 2012 Elsevier Inc. All rights reserved.

review presents data and methods from observational, experimental, and interventional studies corroborating the impact of stress on wound healing. Potential behavioral and physiologic mechanisms explaining the association between stress and impaired wound healing are also discussed.

OBSERVATIONAL STUDIES

Prospective studies examining wound healing–related complications following surgery provide evidence for the impact of stress on wound repair. Greater fear or distress before surgery has been associated with poorer outcomes including longer hospital stays, more postoperative complications, and higher rates of rehospitalization.[2,3] For example, among 111 patients undergoing gallstone removal surgery, those who reported more stress on the third postoperative day had a longer hospital stay, compared with less anxious individuals.[4] Among 309 consenting consecutive patients who underwent an elective coronary artery bypass graft surgery, patients who were more optimistic were less likely to be re-hospitalized than less optimistic individuals. Conversely, patients who experienced more depressive symptoms were more likely to require rehospitalization for infection-related complications than individuals reporting less distress.[5] This result was replicated in a study of 72 patients undergoing coronary artery bypass surgery. Patient who had more depressive symptoms at discharge had more infections and poorer wound healing in the following 6 weeks after surgery than participants who reported less distress.[6]

Psychological factors can also modulate healing of chronic wounds. Fifty-three older adults with chronic lower leg wounds were followed longitudinally to assess speed of wound repair. Patients who experienced the highest levels of depression and anxiety (based on a median split of the Hospital Anxiety and Depression Scale) were 4 times more likely to be categorized in the delayed healing group than individuals who reported less distress.[7] Of importance, in these observational studies distress predicted wound-healing outcomes over and above differences in sociodemographic variables and medical status. Psychological distress thus appears to influence recovery from medical procedures and healing of chronic wounds in clinical settings.

EXPERIMENTAL STUDIES

Animal and human studies in which standard wounds are created experimentally and healing is closely monitored over time provide the strongest evidence of the impact of stress on wound repair. Three main wounding methodologies have been used to study the effect of stress on wound healing.

Punch Biopsy Model

Punch biopsies are used to create standard full-thickness dermal wounds as well as mucosal wounds. Daily pictures of the wound allow for a quantification of changes in wound size over time.

The first human experimental study that examined the impact of stress on wound healing involved family dementia caregivers. Caregivers have to deal daily with the loss of memory, inappropriate emotions, and wandering and restless behavior of their loved ones. Caregiving stress has been associated with heightened anxiety and depression, immune dysregulation, increased risk for cardiovascular disorders, and even death.[8] Family dementia caregiving thus represents an excellent model of chronic stress in humans. A 3.5-mm punch biopsy wound was created on the nondominant forearm of 13 women caregivers and 13 sociodemographically similar noncaregiving controls. Caregivers took 24% longer to heal the small, standardized dermal wound than matched controls, providing initial evidence that chronic stress can delay wound repair.[9]

Stress can also impede healing of a punch biopsy wound among younger people who experienced less intense stress. Twenty-four healthy young men were followed for 21 days after a standard 4-mm punch biopsy was performed on their forearm. In that study, wound healing was assessed using ultrasound biomicroscopy. Stress levels were measured using a self-report questionnaire, the Perceived Stress Scale. Higher perceived stress on the day of the biopsy was associated with slower wound healing.[10] A substantial correlation of -0.59 was found between perceived stress and healing progress between the days 7 and 21 after the biopsy.[10]

Pain, a physical and psychological stressor, can also influence wound healing. A 2-mm full-thickness wound was placed on the back of one upper arm of obese women before receiving elective gastric bypass surgery. Greater acute pain immediately after surgery and persistent pain in the 4 weeks following surgery were associated with slower healing of the experimental wound.[11] Pain generates psychological distress and, when compounded by the presence of other stressors, can put a person at increased risk for delayed wound repair.[12]

Well-controlled animal studies corroborate the impact of stress on wound healing observed in humans. Mice subjected to restraint stress healed a standardized 3.5-mm full-thickness punch biopsy wound on average of 27% more slowly than control mice who were not exposed to the stressor.[13] Restraint stress was also associated with delayed wound healing in a reptilian species, *Urosaurus ornatus* (tree lizard).[14] Social stressors can also impair wound healing. Monogamous California mice, *Peromyscus californicus*, healed a punch biopsy wound more slowly when stressed by the separation from their conspecifics, compared with when they were continuously housed with their conspecifics.[15]

Like cutaneous wounds, mucosal wound healing is also responsive to psychological stress, as demonstrated by a study with academic examination stress. Using a within-subject design, 11 dental students had a biopsy performed on their hard palate during their summer vacation and again 3 days before a major examination. Mucosal wounds placed before the examination healed on average 40% more slowly than identical wounds made during summer vacation. Of importance, the differences in the rate of healing were very consistent: no student healed as rapidly during examinations as during vacation.[16]

The impact of negative emotions on mucosal wound healing was replicated in a larger study. Among 193 healthy undergraduate students who received a 3.5-mm wound on the hard palate, individuals reporting high levels of depressive symptoms were almost 3.6 times more likely to be classified as slow healers than less dysphoric students.[17]

Blister Wounds Model

The blister wounds model is another experimental paradigm designed to study the impact of psychological factors on wound healing. Blister wounds are produced by the application of a vacuum pump on the forearm. A gentle suction creates a separation of the epidermis from the dermis over the course of 1 hour. One of the strengths of this method is that it allows for the collection of data on cytokine production at the wound site, as described below. In this model, wound healing is assessed via measurement of the rate of transepidermal water loss (TEWL). One of the main functions of the skin is to limit movement of water in and out of the body. The permeability of the epidermis increases after the blister wound, but decreases as the healing process unfolds. A computerized evaporimetry instrument can measure vapor pressure gradient in the air layers close to the skin surface. TEWL measurement is a noninvasive means to monitor changes in the stratum corneum barrier function of the skin that provides an excellent objective method for the evaluation of wound healing.

Using a blister wounds paradigm, the discussion of a marital disagreement, a commonplace stressor, delayed wound repair. Married couples were invited for two 24-hour admissions at a hospital research unit. During both visits, 8 8-mm suction blisters were created on the participants' nondominant forearm. Wound healing was monitored for 14 days using TEWL measurements. During the first admission, couples participated in a structured social support interaction task. During the second visit, couples were asked to discuss marital disagreements during a 30-minute period. After both interaction tasks, couples remained in the research unit until the next morning to allow for cytokine measurements and to minimize external influences on wound healing.[18]

Couples' blister wounds healed more slowly following the marital conflict visit than after the social support visit, suggesting that the stress induced by the discussion of marital disagreements interfered with wound repair. Furthermore, the quality of the discussion also influenced the rate of healing. Couples who had more hostile and negative interactions across both the support and the conflict discussions healed wounds more slowly than couples whose interactions were less negative. The overall differences related to hostility were substantial. The blister wounds in high hostile couples healed at only 60% of the rate of low hostile couples.[18]

In a different subset of participants from the same study, positive behaviors during the social support task were also related to wound repair. Individuals who displayed more self-disclosure, acceptance of their partner, relationship-enhancing statements, and humor during the interaction task healed the blister wounds faster than participants who exhibited less positive behaviors during the marital interaction task.[19]

Difficulties in managing one's anger has also been associated with impaired wound healing. Blister wounds were created on the forearm of 98 community-dwelling participants who were followed for 14 days to monitor healing speed. Anger management styles were assessed via a self-report questionnaire, the Spielberger Anger Expression Scale. Participants who had difficulty controlling the expression of their anger were 4.2 times more likely to be classified as slow healers than individuals who reported better anger control. Furthermore, individuals with anger management issues secreted more cortisol in response to the blistering procedure. The increased glucocorticoid production was in turn related to delayed healing.[20]

Tape Stripping to Disrupt Skin Barrier Function

Another wound-healing model consists of the repeated application of cellophane tape to remove a layer of epidermis cells, causing a disruption of the stratum corneum barrier function of the skin. This procedure affects epidermal permeability. Wound healing is assessed by measuring the rate of recovery of the skin barrier function using TEWL measurements.

Acute laboratory stressors can delay the recovery of skin barrier function following its disruption by tape stripping. Twenty-five women participated in the Trier Social Stress Test (TSST), a psychosical stressor.[21] The TSST, a standardized laboratory stressor with a mock job interview and a mental arithmetic task, induces reliable changes in heart rate, and cortisol and cytokine production, and subjective anxiety responses.[22,23] Skin barrier repair was delayed in women after the TSST as compared with a stress-free period.[21]

This result was replicated in a larger study of 85 healthy young men and women. Individuals who participated in the TSST had a slower recovery of skin barrier function than participants who engaged in a reading control task.[24] Furthermore, positive affect had a protective effect on stress-induced delays in skin barrier recovery. Stressed individuals reporting more positive affect recovered faster from the tape-stripping procedure than stressed participants who had low-trait positive affect.[25]

Academic examination stress affects skin barrier recovery. Twenty-seven professional and medical students underwent a tape stripping procedure on 3 occasions: right after their winter and spring vacations, and during their winter final examination week. Skin barrier recovery was significantly delayed at 3, 6, and 24 hours after tape stripping during the examination period, compared with the 2 vacation periods. Furthermore, students reporting the most stress during the examination period had slower recovery in skin barrier function than participants who experienced less examination-induced stress.[26]

The interpersonal stress associated with the dissolution of a committed marital relationship can impede recovery of the stratum corneum barrier function of the skin. Twenty-eight women who were going through a divorce or a separation and 27 women who reported high levels of marital satisfaction underwent a tape-stripping procedure on both facial cheeks. Socially stressed women had delayed skin barrier recovery at 3 and 24 hours following the tape-stripping procedure, compared with less stressed women.[27]

In animal models, different types of stressors can also impair skin barrier recovery. Three days of immobilization stress delayed skin barrier function recovery even for 7 days, compared with control rats not exposed to the stressor.[28] Social reorganization stress associated with cage transfer also impaired the restoration of skin barrier function in rats.[29] These results converge with human data indicating that psychological stress can disrupt skin barrier recovery.

INTERVENTION STUDIES

Intervention studies that improve healing outcomes by reducing psychological stress provide further evidence of the impact of psychological and behavioral factors in wound repair. Meta-analyses of clinical studies show that behavioral stress management interventions before surgery have been associated with improved postoperative outcomes, including fewer medical complications and shorter hospital stays.[30,31]

Written emotional disclosure interventions can decrease psychological distress, improve self-reported health, enhance aspects of cellular immunity, and decrease health care use.[32] Men were randomized to a written emotional disclosure intervention or a nonintervention control group, and received a punch biopsy on the nondominant forearm. Healing was assessed using ultrasound biomicroscopy on 3 occasions during a 21-day period. Men who participated in the emotional disclosure intervention had smaller wounds than control participants at 14 and 21 days.[33]

A brief relaxation intervention improved the healing process among patients undergoing an elective laparoscopic cholecystectomy. Seventy-five consecutive patients were randomized to receive standard care or standard plus the relaxation intervention. The relaxation intervention consisted of deep breathing, progressive muscle relaxation, and guided imagery. The healing process was measured by evaluating the hydroxyproline concentration at the wound site, a measure of collagen deposition. Patients randomized to the brief relaxation intervention had less perceived stress and greater wound hydroxyproline concentration 7 days post-surgery, as well as less fatigue 30 days post-surgery, compared to patients who received the usual care only.[34,35]

Physical exercise can reduce psychological distress in addition to improving cardiovascular function.[36] Older adults were randomized to an exercise intervention

(1-hour aerobic exercise session, 3 times per week) or a nonintervention control group. One month after the beginning of the intervention, participants received a 3.5-mm punch biopsy on the back of their nondominant upper arm. Older adults who exercised healed their wounds faster than those in the control group.[37] In accord with these human data, older mice randomized to a 30-minute daily exercise period during 8 days healed a punch biopsy wound faster than sedentary control mice.[38]

Social support is associated with better health outcomes.[39] In animal studies, monogamous rodents who were housed in pairs healed a standard punch biopsy wound faster than rodents housed alone.[40] Pair housing also buffered the impact of restraint stress on wound healing. Immobilization stress impaired cutaneous wound healing in Siberian hamsters housed alone, but not in hamsters housed in pairs.[41] These data indicate that the presence of a familial conspecific improves wound-healing outcomes in monogamous rodents.

A pharmacologic agent commonly used in the treatment of mood and anxiety disorders is fluoxetine.[42] In a study using alternating isolation and crowding stress, stressed Wistar rats who received fluoxetine healed at a similar pace as their nonstress counterparts, and faster than stressed animals who received only a vehicle injection.[43] These results indicate that pharmacologic stress reduction may also improve wound healing.

In summary, a wide array of acute and chronic stressors can disrupt the healing process. Furthermore, the impact of stress on wound repair has been observed across different methodologies and with different healing outcomes, and most results have replicated in at least 2 independent laboratories. Results from observation, experimental, and intervention studies collectively provide strong evidence that psychological stress can influence wound healing.

BIOLOGY OF WOUND HEALING

A brief review of the biology of wound healing is presented to highlight the pathways by which psychological stress can impede the repair process. Wound healing progresses through several overlapping stages.[44] In the initial inflammatory stage, vasoconstriction and blood coagulation are followed by platelet activation and the release of platelet-derived growth factors (PDGFs) as well as chemoattractant factors released by injured parenchymal cells. Cytokines and chemokines, such as interleukin (IL)-1α, IL-1β, transforming growth factor-β (TGF-β), vascular endothelial growth factor, tumor necrosis factor-α (TNF-α), and IL-8 play important roles in the early stage of wound healing. These factors act as chemoattractants for the migration of phagocytes and other cells to the site, starting the proliferative phase that involves the recruitment and replication of cells necessary for tissue regeneration and capillary regrowth. The final step, wound remodeling, may continue for weeks or months. Thus, the healing process is a cascade, and success in the later stages of wound repair is highly dependent on initial events.[44]

Inflammation plays a key role early in this cascade, and proinflammatory cytokines are essential to this effort; they help to protect against infection and prepare injured tissue for repair by enhancing the recruitment and activation of phagocytes.[43] Furthermore, cytokines released by recruited cells regulate the ability of fibroblasts and epithelial cells to remodel the damaged tissue.[45] IL-1 produced early after tissue injury can regulate the production, release, and activation of metalloproteinases that are important in the destruction and remodeling of the wound; IL-1 also regulates fibroblast chemotaxis and the production of collagen.[45] Moreover, IL-1 stimulates the production of other cytokines that are important for wound healing, including IL-2, IL-6, and IL-8.[45] Confirming the importance of proinflammatory cytokines in the

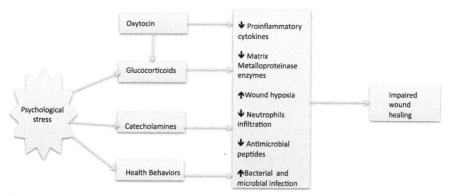

Fig. 1. Behavioral and physiologic pathways linking psychological stress and wound healing.

healing process, IL-6 knock-out mice healed a standard wound 3 times more slowly than wild-type mice.[46] Accordingly, deficits early in the wound repair cascade can have adverse downstream consequences.

PHYSIOLOGIC PATHWAYS OF THE STRESS-INDUCED WOUND-HEALING IMPAIRMENT

Psychological stress leads to the activation of the hypothalamic-pituitary-adrenal and the sympathetic-adrenal-medullary axes.[47] Enhanced glucocorticoids and catecholamines production can directly influence several components of the healing process. Substantial evidence from animal and humans studies indicate that physiologic stress responses can retard the initial inflammatory phase of wound healing.[48] **Fig. 1** presents a schematic representation of the behavioral and physiologic pathways linking stress and wound healing.

Glucocorticoids

Stress-induced glucocorticoid production has been associated with delayed wound healing. In humans, greater awakening cortisol secretion the day following a punch biopsy was associated with greater perceived stress and delayed wound healing.[10] In animal studies, restraint stress led to a fourfold elevation in corticosterone levels.[13] Blocking glucocorticoid function with a glucocorticoid receptor antagonist, RU40555, eliminated the stress-induced delay in wound healing in stressed animals.[13,41] Preventing glucocorticoid production via adrenalectomy also reduced the effects of restraint stress on wound healing.[41] Furthermore, exogenous administration of glucocorticoid slowed wound healing as compared with a vehicle injection.[13]

Catecholamines

Increased catecholamine production also appears to play a role in stress-induced impairment in wound healing. Administration of an α-adrenergic receptor antagonist attenuated the restraint stress-induced impairment of wound healing in mice.[49] In a study using a rotation stress model, administration of a β-adrenergic receptor antagonist, propranolol hydrochloride, attenuated the stress-induced impairment in wound healing in mice.[50] In a burn wound model, mice injected with a β-adrenergic receptor antagonist exhibited improved reepithelialization of burn wounds, compared with mice who received a vehicle injection.[51] Furthermore, injection of norepinephrine can reduce keratinocyte motility and migration in vitro.[51] These data provide evidence of a role for catecholamines in stress-induced impairment in wound repair.

Oxytocin and Vasopressin

The two hypothalamic peptides, oxytocin and vasopressin, modulated physiologic stress responses and social bonding processes in animal and human work. In a couples study using the blister wounds model, individuals who had more positive interactions with their partner during a social support task had higher plasma oxytocin levels. Higher circulating oxytocin levels were in turn associated with faster healing of the standard blister wounds. Furthermore, in women, but not in men, greater plasma vasopressin levels were related to faster healing.[19]

Well-controlled animal studies corroborate the role of oxytocin in mediating the beneficial effects of social relationships on wound healing. Exogenous oxytocin administration attenuated the stress-induced corticosterone production and impairment in wound healing.[41,52] Furthermore, administration of an oxytocin receptor antagonist eliminated the beneficial impact of pair housing on wound healing.[41] These results collectively suggest that in addition to modulating stress responses, oxytocin may have a direct influence on the healing process.

Local Cytokine Production

Diminished expression of proinflammatory cytokines at the wound site is another pathway by which stress can delay the initial phase of wound healing. The suction blister model provides a method to monitor in vivo cytokine expression at the wound site in humans. After raising several blisters and removing their roofs (the epidermis), plastic templates with wells containing a salt solution and autologous serum are placed over the lesions to monitor protein expression at the wound site. The autologous serum-buffer solution is aspirated from the wells with a syringe at different time intervals, allowing for cell phenotyping and cytokine measurement as the local immune response evolves.

Using this approach, women who reported more perceived stress produced significantly lower IL-1α and IL-8 levels at the wound site, 5 and 24 hours after the blistering procedure.[53] Marital disagreement also influenced local cytokine production.[18] Production of three proinflammatory cytokines at the wound site, IL-1β, IL-6, and TNF-α, were lower after the discussion of a marital disagreement than after a social support discussion, paralleling the impact of marital conflict on wound healing.[18] In these two studies, local cytokine production was not significantly associated with serum levels of the same cytokines, underscoring the different biologic significance of local and systemic production of these molecules.

In a clinical study, patients undergoing surgery for hernia removal who reported greater preoperative stress had a lower concentration of IL-1β in the wound drain fluid 20 hours after the operation, compared with patients who experienced less preoperative distress.[54] Furthermore, two stressors that can impair cutaneous and mucosal wound healing, family dementia caregiving and academic examinations, were also associated with poorer stimulated production of IL-1β after treatment with lipopolysaccharide.[9,16] Corroborating human data, mice subjected to restraint stress had lower levels of IL-1β mRNA at the wound site, compared with control mice.[55,56]

Stress-induced glucocorticoid production might effectively decrease cytokine production at the wound site. Exogenous administration of glucocorticoid diminished IL-1α, IL-1β, and TNF-α expression at the site after wounding in mice.[44] Similarly, animal and human studies have also demonstrated that stress-induced elevations in glucocorticoids can transiently suppress IL-1β, TNF-α, and PDGF production.[53,56]

Accordingly, dysregulation of glucocorticoid secretion provides one obvious neuroendocrine pathway through which stress alters the initial inflammatory phase of wound healing.

Matrix Metalloproteinase

Matrix metalloproteinase (MMP) enzymes are involved in the degradation of collagen and other extracellular matrix molecules. Degradation of the basement membrane of the wound promotes cellular invasion and migration, an essential component of the early phase of wound healing. Among patients undergoing inguinal hernia surgery, those who reported greater worry about the operation had lower levels of MMP-9 in the wound drain fluid 20 hours after surgery.[54] In a human study using the blister wounds model, there was a negative correlation between plasma cortisol levels and MMP-2 protein levels at the wound site.[57] Furthermore, in an animal study using a rotation stress model, mice subjected to the stressor had fewer activated MMP-2 and MMP-9 7 days after wounding, compared with control mice.[50] These data indicate that stress can downregulate MMP production at the wound site.

Wound Cellularity

Psychological stress may reduce cell infiltration at the wound site. In a study using a restraint stress paradigm, cellularity of the wound and wound margin areas were analyzed in cross sections of dermal and epidermal layers. Mice subjected to restraint stress had less leukocyte infiltration to the wound sites than control mice at 1 and 3 days after wounding.[13]

Increased Susceptibility to Infection

Stress can also increase susceptibility to wound infection. Mice exposed to restraint stress had a 2- to 5-log increase in opportunistic bacteria such as *Staphylococcus aureus*, compared with control mice not exposed to the stressor. Furthermore, 7 days after wounding, 85.4% of restraint-stress mice had bacterial counts predictive of infection, compared with 27.4% of controls.[58]

The increased susceptibility to infection appears to be mediated in part by a decreased epidermal antimicrobial peptides production. Mice exposed to insomnia and crowding stress had lower epidermis levels of cathelin-related antimicrobial peptides and exhibited more severe infection following an intradermal injection of group A *Streptococcus pyogenes*.[59] This effect appears to be glucocorticoid dependent; administration of a glucocorticoid receptor antagonist eliminated the impact of stress on epidermis antimicrobial peptide production, and administration of exogenous glucocorticoid mimicked the effects of stress on antimicrobial production.[59]

Wound Hypoxia

Oxygen homeostasis is critical to all phases of wound healing. Damage created to blood vessels during wounding decreases oxygen availability. Simultaneously, neutrophils' oxidative burst increases oxygen demand at the wound site. Restraint stress can further promote wound hypoxia.[60] Compared with controls, restraint-stressed mice had higher levels of inducible nitric oxide synthase levels, an indicator of wound hypoxia at the wound site.[60] Furthermore, hyperbaric oxygen therapy normalized inducible nitric oxide synthase levels and attenuated stress-induced impairments in wound healing.[60]

BEHAVIORAL MECHANISMS LINKING STRESS AND WOUND HEALING

In addition to directly modulating physiologic responses to skin damage, stress can also indirectly influence wound repair by promoting the adoption of health-damaging behaviors. Individuals who experience greater levels of stress are more likely to increase their alcohol and tobacco use, decrease their participation in physical activity, experience sleep disturbances, and make poorer diet choices than individuals reporting less distress.[61,62] These negative health behavior practices can then compound the detrimental impact of stress on physiologic healing processes.[2]

Heavy alcohol use has been associated with delays in cell migration and collagen deposition at the wound site, which in turn can impede the healing process.[63] Smoking has also been related to slowed healing of naturally occurring and surgical wounds.[64] Sleep disruption delays skin barrier recovery after tape stripping and diminishes growth hormone production.[21,65] Lack of regular physical activity can slow the rate of wound healing.[38] Furthermore, deficient intake of glucose, polyunsaturated proteins, and certain vitamins can impede the healing process.[66–68]

SUMMARY

The goal of this review is to present clinical and experimental models of the impact of stress on wound repair. Converging and replicated evidence from experimental and clinical models of wound healing indicates that psychological stress leads to clinically relevant delays in wound healing. New mechanistic data suggest ways to elucidate the multiple physiologic pathways by which stress alters wound repair processes. Translational work should focus on identifying conditions in which behavioral and pharmacologic treatments are the most effective and on developing new treatments able to attenuate stress-induced delays in wound healing.

REFERENCES

1. Walburn J, Vedhara K, Hankins M, et al. Psychological stress and wound healing in humans: a systematic review and meta-analysis. J Psychosom Res 2009;67(3):253–71.
2. Kiecolt-Glaser JK, Page GG, Marucha PT, et al. Psychological influences on surgical recovery: perspectives from psychoneuroimmunology. Am Psychol 1998;53:1209–18.
3. Rosenberger PH, Jokl P, Ickovics J. Psychosocial factors and surgical outcomes: an evidence-based literature review. J Am Acad Orthop Surg 2006;14(7):397–405.
4. Boeke S, Duivenvoorden HJ, Verhage F, et al. Prediction of postoperative pain and duration of hospitalization using two anxiety measures. Pain 1991;45(3):293–7.
5. Scheier MF, Matthews KA, Owens JF, et al. Optimism and rehospitalization after coronary artery bypass graft surgery. Arch Intern Med 1999;159:829–35.
6. Doering LV, Moser DK, Lemankiewicz W, et al. Depression, healing, and recovery from coronary artery bypass surgery. Am J Crit Care 2005;14(4):316–24.
7. Cole-King A, Harding KG. Psychological factors and delayed healing in chronic wounds. Psychosom Med 2001;63:216–20.
8. Gouin JP, Hantsoo L, Kiecolt-Glaser JK. Immune dysregulation and chronic stress among older adults: a review. Neuroimmunomodulation 2008;15(4–6):251–9.
9. Kiecolt-Glaser JK, Marucha PT, Malarkey WB, et al. Slowing of wound healing by psychological stress. Lancet 1995;346:1194–6.
10. Ebrecht M, Hextall J, Kirtley LG, et al. Perceived stress and cortisol levels predict speed of wound heating in healthy male adults. Psychoneuroendocrinology 2004; 29(6):798–809.
11. McGuire L, Heffner K, Glaser R, et al. Pain and wound healing in surgical patients. Ann Behav Med 2006;31(2):165–72.

12. Graham JE, Robles TF, Kiecolt-Glaser JK, et al. Hostility and pain are related to inflammation in older adults. Brain Behav Immun 2006;20(4):389–400.
13. Padgett DA, Marucha PT, Sheridan JF. Restraint stress slows cutaneous wound healing in mice. Brain Behav Immun 1998;12:64–73.
14. French SS, Matt KS, Moore MC. The effects of stress on wound healing in male tree lizards (Urosaurus ornatus). Gen Comp Endocrinol 2006;145(2):128–32.
15. Martin LB 2nd, Glasper ER, Nelson RJ, et al. Prolonged separation delays wound healing in monogamous California mice, Peromyscus californicus, but not in polygynous white-footed mice, P. leucopus. Physiol Behav 2006;87(5):837–41.
16. Marucha PT, Kiecolt-Glaser JK, Favagehi M. Mucosal wound healing is impaired by examination stress. Psychosom Med 1998;60:362–5.
17. Bosch JA, Engeland CG, Cacioppo JT, et al. Depressive symptoms predict mucosal wound healing. Psychosom Med 2007;69(7):597–605.
18. Kiecolt-Glaser JK, Loving TJ, Stowell JR, et al. Hostile marital interactions, proinflammatory cytokine production, and wound healing. Arch Gen Psychiatry 2005;62:1377–84.
19. Gouin JP, Carter CS, Pournajafi-Nazarloo H, et al. Marital behavior, oxytocin, vasopressin, and wound healing. Psychoneuroendocrinology 2010;35(7):1082–90.
20. Gouin JP, Kiecolt-Glaser JK, Malarkey WB, et al. The influence of anger expression on wound healing. Brain Behav Immun 2008;22(5):699–708.
21. Altemus M, Rao B, Dhabhar FS, et al. Stress-induced changes in skin barrier function in healthy women. J Invest Dermatol 2001;117:309–17.
22. Dickerson SS, Kemeny ME. Acute stressors and cortisol responses: a theoretical integration and synthesis of laboratory research. Psychol Bull 2004;130(3):355–91.
23. Kirschbaum C, Pirke KM, Hellhammer DH. The "Trier social stress test"—a tool for investigating psychobiological stress responses in a laboratory setting. Neuropsychobiology 1993;28:76–81.
24. Robles TF. Stress, social support, and delayed skin barrier recovery. Psychosom Med 2007;69(8):807–15.
25. Robles TF, Brooks KP, Pressman SD. Trait positive affect buffers the effects of acute stress on skin barrier recovery. Health Psychol 2009;28(3):373–8.
26. Garg A, Chren MM, Sands LP, et al. Psychological stress perturbs epidermal permeability barrier homeostasis: implications for the pathogenesis of stress-associated skin disorders. Arch Dermatol 2000;137:53–9.
27. Muizzuddin N, Matsui MS, Marenus KD, et al. Impact of stress of marital dissolution on skin barrier recovery: tape stripping and measurement of trans-epidermal water loss (TEWL). Skin Res Technol 2003;9:34–8.
28. Denda M, Tsuchiya T, Hosoi J, et al. Immobilization-induced and crowded environment-induced stress delay barrier recovery in murine skin. Br J Dermatol 1998;138:780–5.
29. Denda M, Tsuchiya T, Elias PM, et al. Stress alters cutaneous permeability barrier homeostasis. Am J Physiol Regul Integr Comp Physiol 2000;278:R367–72.
30. Johnston M, Vogele C. Benefits of psychological preparation for surgery: a meta-analysis. Ann Behav Med 1993;15:245–56.
31. Montgomery GH, David D, Winkel G, et al. The effectiveness of adjunctive hypnosis with surgical patients: a meta-analysis. Anesth Analg 2002;94(6):1639–45.
32. Esterling BA, L'Abate L, Murray EJ, et al. Empirical foundations for writing in prevention and psychotherapy: mental and physical health outcomes. Clin Psychol Rev 1999;19(1):79–96.
33. Weinman J, Ebrecht M, Scott S, et al. Enhanced wound healing after emotional disclosure intervention. Br J Health Psychol 2008;13(Pt 1):95–102.

34. Broadbent E, Kahoekehr A, Booth RJ, et al. A brief relaxation intervention reduces stress and improves surgical wound healing response: a randomized trial. Brain Behav Immun 2012;26(2):212–7.
35. Kahoekehr A, Broadbent E, Wheeler BR, et al. The effect of perioperative psychological intervention on fatigue after laparoscopic cholecystectomy: a randomized controlled trial. Surg Endosc 2012. [Epub ahead of print].
36. Emery CF, Blumenthal JA, Glaser R, et al. Effects of physical exercise on psychological and cognitive functioning of older adults. Ann Behav Med 1991;13:99–107.
37. Emery CF, Kiecolt-Glaser JK, Glaser R, et al. Exercise accelerates wound healing among healthy older adults: a preliminary investigation. J Gerontol A Biol Sci Med Sci 2005;60(11):1432–6.
38. Keylock KT, Vieira VJ, Wallig MA, et al. Exercise accelerates cutaneous wound healing and decreases wound inflammation in aged mice. Am J Physiol Regul Integr Comp Physiol 2008;294(1):R179–84.
39. House JS, Landis KR, Umberson D. Social relationships and health. Science 1988; 241:540–5.
40. Glasper ER, Devries AC. Social structure influences effects of pair-housing on wound healing. Brain Behav Immun 2005;19(1):61–8.
41. Detillion CE, Craft TK, Glasper ER, et al. Social facilitation of wound healing. Psychoneuroendocrinology 2004;29(8):1004–11.
42. Rossi A, Barraco A, Donda P. Fluoxetine: a review on evidence based medicine. Ann Gen Hosp Psychiatry 2004;3(1):2.
43. Farahani RM, Sadr K, Rad JS, et al. Fluoxetine enhances cutaneous wound healing in chronically stressed Wistar rats. Adv Skin Wound Care 2007;20(3):157–65.
44. Hubner G, Brauchle M, Smola H, et al. Differential regulation of pro-inflammatory cytokines during wound healing in normal glucocorticoid-treated mice. Cytokine 1996;8(7):548–56.
45. Werner S, Grose R. Regulation of wound healing by growth factors and cytokines. Physiol Rev 2003;83(3):835–70.
46. Gallucci RM, Simeonova PP, Matheson JM, et al. Impaired cutaneous wound healing in interleukin-6-deficient and immunosuppressed mice. FASEB J 2000;14:2525–31.
47. Padgett DA, Glaser R. How stress influences the immune response. Trends Immunol 2003;24(8):444–8.
48. Glaser R, Kiecolt-Glaser JK. Stress-induced immune dysfunction: implications for health. Nat Rev Immunol 2005;5:243–51.
49. Eijkelkamp N, Engeland CG, Gajendrareddy PK, et al. Restraint stress impairs early wound healing in mice via alpha-adrenergic but not beta-adrenergic receptors. Brain Behav Immun 2007;21(4):409–12.
50. Romana-Souza B, Otranto M, Vieira AM, et al. Rotational stress-induced increase in epinephrine levels delays cutaneous wound healing in mice. Brain Behav Immun 2010;24(3):427–37.
51. Sivamani RK, Pullar CE, Manabat-Hidalgo CG, et al. Stress-mediated increases in systemic and local epinephrine impair skin wound healing: potential new indication for beta blockers. PLoS Med 2009;6(1):e12.
52. Vitalo A, Fricchione J, Casali M, et al. Nest making and oxytocin comparably promote wound healing in isolation reared rats. PLoS One 2009;4(5):e5523.
53. Glaser R, Kiecolt-Glaser JK, Marucha PT, et al. Stress-related changes in proinflammatory cytokine production in wounds. Arch Gen Psychiatry 1999;56:450–6.
54. Broadbent E, Petrie KJ, Alley PG, et al. Psychological stress impairs early wound repair following surgery. Psychosom Med 2003;65(5):865–9.

55. Mercado AM, Padgett DA, Sheridan JF, et al. Altered kinetics of IL-1 alpha, IL-1 beta, and KGF-1 gene expression in early wounds of restrained mice. Brain Behav Immun 2002;16(2):150–62.

56. Head CC, Farrow MJ, Sheridan JF, et al. Androstenediol reduces the anti-inflammatory effects of restraint stress during wound healing. Brain Behav Immun 2006;20(6):590–6.

57. Yang EV, Bane CM, MacCallum RC, et al. Stress-related modulation of matrix metalloproteinase expression. J Neuroimmunol 2002;133(1-2):144–50.

58. Rojas I, Padgett DA, Sheridan JF, et al. Stress-induced susceptibility to bacterial infection during cutaneous wound healing. Brain Behav Immun 2002;16:74–84.

59. Aberg KM, Radek KA, Choi EH, et al. Psychological stress downregulates epidermal antimicrobial peptide expression and increases severity of cutaneous infections in mice. J Clin Invest 2007;117(11):3339–49.

60. Gajendrareddy PK, Sen CK, Horan MP, et al. Hyperbaric oxygen therapy ameliorates stress-impaired dermal wound healing. Brain Behav Immun 2005;19(3):217–22.

61. Steptoe A, Wardle J, Pollard TM, et al. Stress, social support and health-related behavior: a study of smoking, alcohol consumption and physical exercise. J Psychosom Res 1996;41:171–80.

62. Vitaliano PP, Scanlan JM, Zhang J, et al. A path model of chronic stress, the metabolic syndrome, and coronary heart disease. Psychosom Med 2002;64:418–35.

63. Benveniste K, Thut P. The effect of chronic alcoholism on wound healing. Proc Soc Exp Biol Med 1981;166:568–75.

64. Silverstein P. Smoking and wound healing. Am J Med 1992;93:22S–4S.

65. Veldhuis JD, Iranmanesch A. Physiological regulation of the human growth hormone (GH)-insulin-like growth factor type I (IGF-I) axis: predominant impact of age, obesity, gonadal function, and sleep. Sleep 1996;19:S221–4.

66. Russell L. The importance of patients' nutritional status in wound healing. Br J Nurs 2001;10(6 Suppl):S42, S44–9.

67. Posthauer ME. The role of nutrition in wound care. Adv Skin Wound Care 2006;19(1):43–52 [quiz: 53–4].

68. McDaniel JC, Belury M, Ahijevych K, et al. Omega-3 fatty acids effect on wound healing. Wound Repair Regen 2008;16(3):337–45.

Wound Management

Maria E. Moreira, MD[a],*, Vincent J. Markovchick, MD[a,b,c]

KEYWORDS

- Wounds • Lacerations • Wound management

KEY POINTS

- Wound management makes up an important part of the emergency physician's practice. Understanding the physiology of wound healing and both patient and wound factors affecting this process is essential for the proper treatment of wounds.
- Though there are many options available for wound closure, the choice of closure needs to be appropriate for the wound.
- Each modality has its benefits and its drawbacks and some are only appropriate for certain types of wounds. The goal is to achieve the best functional and cosmetically appealing scar while avoiding complications.

Management of traumatic wounds is one of the most common procedures practiced in emergency medicine representing approximately 8 percent of emergency department (ED) presentations.[1] It is the most visible manifestation of emergency practice, in that the result of the physician's efforts is with the patient for their entire life. Wound care practices, however, have been based mostly on experience with a paucity of well-performed, randomized, controlled clinical trials to support these practices.

There has been controversy over different aspects of wound care including timing of wound closure, the best method of wound closure, the preparation of wounds, and antibiotic use in traumatic wounds. Studies relevant to these aspects of wound management are discussed further in this article. The article also discusses future innovative methods for wound management including the use of botulinum toxin, hyaluronidase injections, and porcine small intestinal submucosa (SIS). Emergency medicine physicians strive to provide patients with the best care in a timely fashion based on the current evidence. In wound management, this goal translates to providing painless, quick wound closure with an excellent cosmetic result and avoiding infection. New methods of wound closure that meet all these criteria are discussed.

[a] Department of Emergency Medicine, University of Colorado School of Medicine, 777 Bannock Street, Mailcode 0108, Denver, CO 80204, USA; [b] Emergency Medical Services, Denver Health, 777 Bannock Street, MC 0108, Denver, CO 80204, USA; [c] Denver Health Medical Center, Denver, CO, USA
* Corresponding author.
E-mail address: maria.moreira@dhha.org

Crit Care Nurs Clin N Am 24 (2012) 215–237
doi:10.1016/j.ccell.2012.03.008
0899-5885/12/$ – see front matter © 2012 Elsevier Inc. All rights reserved.

PHYSIOLOGY

The goal in wound management is an ideal functional or cosmetic result without any complication. To achieve this goal, the clinician must have a basic understanding of wound physiology and factors that potentially can affect normal wound healing.

When wounding occurs, wound edges retract, and tissue contracts. Subsequently platelets aggregate on the exposed wound surface, the clotting cascade is activated, and a hemostatic coagulum is formed. The inflammatory response follows with granulocytes and lymphocytes migrating to the wound helping to control bacterial growth and suppress infection. Macrophages are the predominant cell present in the wound by day 5. These cells play a role in early fibroblast and collagen formation. As the inflammatory response evolves, epithelial cells form pseudopod-like structures and move over the wound surface. After laceration repair, initial epithelialization occurs within 24 to 48 hours. Peak synthesis of collagen occurs between days 5 and 7. Because of the balance between synthesis and lysis, however, there is a vulnerable period between days 7 and 10 after initial injury when wounds are prone to dehiscence. The wound will be at 5% of its ultimate tensile strength at 2 weeks and at about 35% at 1 month.[2]

CLINICAL EVALUATION
History

A thorough history is paramount for discerning host factors affecting wound healing. Multiple patient conditions have been shown to increase the risk of infection. These conditions include extremes of age, diabetes mellitus, chronic renal failure, obesity, malnutrition, and inherited or acquired connective tissue disorders.[3] The use of certain medications is important also. Immunosuppressive medications such as corticosteroids have been shown to affect wound healing negatively and to increase the potential for infection.[3]

Wound and environmental factors also contribute to wound healing. The clinician needs to ascertain if the wound was caused by a cut or by blunt trauma. Compressive forces as the mechanism of injury increase the risk for infection because of compromised circulation to the wound edges.[4] Retained foreign bodies increase the risk of an inflammatory response and subsequent infection and abscess formation. A "dirty" wound may or may not be a "contaminated" wound. Contaminated wounds are those in which there is a high degree of bacterial inoculation at the time of wounding. Mechanisms include mammalian bites, human bites, and wounds incurred in submerged bodies of water (eg, streams, lakes, ponds). Also "old" wounds should be considered contaminated because of the high level of bacteria 6 to 8 hours after wounding.

The time from injury to evaluation can affect the type of closure performed. The concept of the "golden period" stems from the assumption that bacterial proliferation within wounds is dependent on time from initial insult to repair. All wounds, including "clean" wounds, have bacteria introduced at the time of wounding. Although bacteria are in the wound at the time of presentation,[5,6] however, most wounds have bacterial counts well below the infectious inoculum of 10^5 or more organisms per gram.[6] A period of 3 to 5 hours generally is required for proliferation of bacteria to produce infection,[6] and after 8 hours the bacterial count rises exponentially.

A study undertaken in Jamaica suggested a 19-hour golden period for the repair of simple wounds in areas other than the head. Wounds sutured after 19 hours were less likely to heal. Healing of wounds involving the head was unaffected by the interval between injury and repair.[7] This study quotes time periods slightly longer than the standard period suggested for the interval before extremity wound closure. The accepted interval from injury to wound closure is up to 6 hours for wounds to the extremities and up to 24 hours for face and scalp wounds.

Some clinicians suggest that timing is not important if the wound is clean and not infected.[8] Each wound needs to be considered individually as to the time and mechanism of injury as well as wound and host characteristics affecting potential functional and cosmetic outcome. The clinician may decide to close a clean leg wound on a healthy patient after 10 hours and not to close a contaminated leg wound on a diabetic after 4 hours.

Other important aspects of the history include allergies to medications and tetanus immunization status. The incidence of tetanus has declined since tetanus toxoid vaccine was introduced in the 1940s. From 1998 to 2000, the average annual incidence of tetanus was 0.16 cases per million population. Most of the cases reported during that time occurred in people who had inadequate vaccination or unknown vaccination history and who sustained an acute injury.[9]

If a patient has an inadequate immunization history or has never been immunized, tetanus immune globulin (250 IU) and tetanus toxoid (0.5 mL) are indicated. A primary series of tetanus toxoid induces protective levels of serum antitoxin persisting for 10 years or longer.[10] Booster for minor and uncontaminated wounds needs to be given only every 10 years. With other wounds, booster should be administered if the patient has not received tetanus toxoid within 5 years. Tetanus-diphtheria toxoid (0.5 mL) is preferred for patients 7 years of age and older, whereas diphtheria, pertussis, and tetanus (0.5 mL) should be used in patients under the age of 7 years. For the patient who has a tetanus-prone wound and unknown tetanus immunization or less than three tetanus toxoid doses, tetanus immune globulin as well as toxoid should be given. Tetanus immune globulin provides passive immunity. If the patient presents with a non–tetanus-prone wound, only toxoid is required. A wound is considered tetanus-prone if it has any of the following features: age of wound greater than 6 hours, stellate wound or avulsion, depth of wound greater than 1 cm, mechanism of injury is a missile, crush, burn or frostbite, signs of infection are present, devitalized tissue is present, presence of contaminants (dirt, feces, soil, or saliva), or presence of denervated or ischemic tissue. If both tetanus immune globulin and toxoid are given, they need to be given in different syringes and at separate sites.

Physical Examination

Proper physical examination and documentation of the wound includes location, length in centimeters, neurovascular examination, motor examination, exploration for tendon or joint involvement, and presence of foreign body. Some wound characteristics noted on physical examination portend a higher rate of infection. In a cross-sectional study of patients who had traumatic lacerations, wound characteristics associated with higher infection rates included jagged wound edges, stellate shape, injury deeper than the subcutaneous tissue, presence of a foreign body, and visible contaminants (ie, dirt and others).[11] Infection was defined as the presence of a stitch abscess, purulent drainage, or cellulites more than 1 cm beyond the wound edges.

A thorough neurovascular examination needs to be performed before anesthetizing the wound. Two-point discrimination at the finger pads provides the best assessment of digital nerve function.[12] Any sensory deficits, problems with motor function, and the presence of pulses or capillary refill need to be documented. If there is a suspicion of a fracture, a radiograph should be obtained before moving a joint through full range of motion. The motor examination provides an evaluation of motor nerves, muscle groups, and tendons.

All wounds need to be explored to evaluate for tendon lacerations and foreign bodies. To obtain optimal examination of the wound, good lighting and a bloodless field are essential. Several methods are available to control bleeding from wounds. Direct external pressure almost always is successful in controlling bleeding. If the wound is in an extremity, and bleeding cannot be controlled with direct external pressure, the next option is to inflate a sphygmomanometer proximal to the site of bleeding. The cuff needs to be inflated to a pressure greater than the patient's systolic blood pressure. The clinician needs to keep track of the time of cuff inflation, which, in general, can be maintained for about 2 hours without producing injury to vessels or nerves. Digital tourniquets, on fingers or toes, should be used only for 20 to 30 minutes at a time.

Because the position of joints and tendons during injury can differ from the position during examination, once a bloodless field is obtained, the depth of the wound needs to be visualized while the extremity is taken through full range of motion. Remember that a tendon can be 90% lacerated and still maintain normal motor function. Avoid motor testing for tendon injury against resistance to prevent from converting a partial tendon laceration into a complete tendon laceration.

It also is important to detect and remove foreign bodies within the wound because the presence of a foreign body poses an increased risk of infection. Other reasons for removal of foreign bodies include impairment of mechanical function, potential for causing persistent pain, and potential for migration. When possible, all foreign bodies should be removed. For those that are minute or deep in tissue or muscle, the risks versus benefits of exploration and removal must be evaluated. If a foreign body does not meet an indication for removal and is not readily accessible, it should be left in place, and the patient must be informed of the risk/benefit assessment and the reason for leaving a retained foreign body in situ.

Careful consideration should be given to handling of tissues when exploring wounds. The clinician must avoid any further damage to the tissue while obtaining a clear visualization of the depth of the wound. Instead of using toothed forceps to grasp wound edges, a nontoothed forcep should be used or alternatively, the forcep should be used to push the edges apart. Skin hooks also can be used to lift wound edges apart. If skin hooks are not available, hooks can be created by bending the tips of a 20-gauge needle.[12]

Diagnostic Evaluation

The use of diagnostic adjuncts is unnecessary for most wounds. Physical examination and exploration after hemorrhage control usually provide a thorough evaluation of the wound. If the wound extends into muscle belly, and the mechanism is compatible with a foreign body (eg, broken glass), radiographs are indicated. Eighty percent to 90% of foreign bodies are detected by radiograph,[13,14] but radiographs may not detect organic foreign bodies such as wood splinters and vegetable matter. In those instances, ultrasound may detect organic foreign bodies not visible on radiographs. CT is the modality of choice for the detection of foreign bodies when other techniques have failed.

THERAPEUTIC INTERVENTION
Anesthesia

Proper wound evaluation, exploration, and closure are enhanced by good anesthesia. Modalities for administration of anesthesia include topical, direct wound infiltration, or regional nerve blocks. Certain patients may require procedural sedation as an adjunct to local anesthesia. In many cases more than one form of anesthesia is beneficial.

Although topical anesthetics decrease the pain of subsequent anesthetic injection, they require time to take effect. Investigators have shown that a topical anesthetic such as 4% lidocaine, 1:2000 epinephrine, and 0.5% tetracaine can be applied effectively by nurses at triage.[15] This administration helps decrease the amount of time from presentation to repair. **Table 1** provides a list of available topical anesthetics and their onset and duration of action.

There are two categories of local anesthetics: the amides and the esters. Allergy to one group is not associated with allergy to anesthetic from the other group. Most allergies are caused by preservatives used in the anesthetic. Therefore, a pure agent such as cardiac lidocaine can be used in patients who have allergies to anesthetics.

The maximum safe dose of an anesthetic must be considered when performing infiltration (**Table 2**). This maximum safe dose increases with the addition of epinephrine to the solution. Epinephrine should be avoided in areas with end arterioles and lack of collateral circulation. These sites include the fingers, toes, the tip of the nose, pinna, and penis.

The pain of local infiltration can be diminished by injecting subcutaneously through the open wound edge instead of directly into intact skin[16,17] with the smallest needle possible. Although 30-gauge needles can be used for direct infiltration, 25- or 27-gauge needles are better suited for regional nerve blocks to decrease the possibility of deflection of the needle.[18] Other available techniques to decrease pain of infiltration include buffering the anesthetic with sodium bicarbonate in a 1:10 solution, using warm solutions, using slow rates of infiltration, and pretreatment with topical anesthetic.[19–21]

Regional anesthesia blocks the nerve supply to the area of the laceration. Regional anesthesia is preferred to local infiltration in three specific situations: (1) in wounds that otherwise would require large, toxic amounts of local anesthetic; (2) in wounds in which local tissue distortion needs to be avoided (eg, lips and digits); (3) in wounds where local infiltration is particularly painful (eg, plantar surface of the foot). In these cases the discomfort of percutaneous injection can be reduced using topical cryotherapy with an ice cube. A further description of regional nerve blocks can be found in any emergency medicine procedural textbook.

Procedural sedation and anesthesia may be required in cases of extensive wound repair, especially in children. The goal is to achieve a depressed level of consciousness while maintaining a patent airway. Procedural sedation can be performed safely and effectively by emergency physicians in both community- and university-based settings. **Table 3** provides a partial list of drugs available for this type of anesthesia [22].

In the pediatric population there has been some emphasis on use of distraction techniques (ie, music, video games, or cartoon videos) to improve satisfaction with wound repair and decrease the stress of wound repair. With distraction, the child's attention is diverted away from the stressful stimulus and focused onto a more pleasant one. Sinha and colleagues[23] found these techniques to be effective in reducing situational anxiety in older children and also in lowering parental perception of pain distress in younger children. Distraction did not reduce self-reported pain intensity, however. The children enrolled in this study had uncomplicated lacerations less than 5 cm in length.

Wound Preparation

Wound preparation is a crucial aspect of wound management that affects infection rate. Saline irrigation decreases the incidence of wound infection in proportion to the amount of irrigation used.[12,24,25] The pressure at which this irrigant is delivered is crucial in determining the efficacy of irrigation.[26,27] With high-pressure irrigation, there is a balance between achieving a reduction in bacterial wound counts and causing further tissue damage. The recommended irrigation pressure is 5 to 8 psi,[18,26,28]

Table 1
Topical anesthetics

Anesthetic Product	Methods	Onset/Duration	Effectiveness	Complications
TAC	2–5 mL (1 mL/cm of laceration) applied to wound with cotton or gauze for 10–30 minutes	Onset: effective 10–30 min after application. Duration: not established.	May be as effective as lidocaine for lacerations on face and scalp	Rare severe toxicity, including seizures and sudden cardiac death
LET	1–3 mL applied directly to wound for 15–30 minutes	Onset: 20–30 min. Duration: not established.	Similar to TAC for face and scalp lacerations; less effective on extremities	No severe adverse effects reported
EMLA	Thick layer (1–2 g/10 cm²) applied to intact skin with covering patch of transparent medical dressing	Onset: must be left on for 1–2 h. Duration: 0.5–2 h	Variable, depending on duration of application	Contact dermatitis, methemoglobinemia (very rare)

Abbreviations: EMLA, 2.5% lidocaine and 2.5% prilocaine; LET, 4% lidocaine, 1:2000 epinephrine, and 0.5% tetracaine; TAC, 0.5% tetracaine, 1:2000 epinephrine, and 11.8% cocaine.
Data from Kundu S, Achar S. Principles of office anesthesia: part II. Topical anesthesia. Am Fam Physician 2002;66:100.

Table 2
Local anesthetics

Agent	Class	Maximum Allowable Single Dose	Onset of Action	Duration of Action
Lidocaine	Amide	4.5 mg/kg of 1%	Fast	1–2 h
Lidocaine with epinephrine	Amide	7 mg/kg of 1%	Fast	2–4 h
Bupivacaine	Amide	2 mg/kg of 0.25%	Intermediate	4–8 h
Bupivacaine with epinephrine	Amide	3 mg/kg of 0.25%	Intermediate	8–16 h
Procaine	Ester	7 mg/kg	Slow	15–45 min
Procaine with epinephrine	Ester	9 mg/kg	Slow	30–60 min

which can be achieved by using a 30- to 60-mL syringe and a 19-gauge needle or splash shield. This pressure also can be obtained by using a saline bag inside a pressure cuff inflated to 400 mm Hg and connected to intravenous tubing with a 19-gauge angiocath[29] or by using a mechanical irrigator. The location of the wound also needs to be considered when determining the irrigation pressure. Although high-pressure irrigation is indicated for contaminated wounds in the extremities, it is not indicated in highly vascularized areas containing loose areolar tissue. High-pressure irrigation of chest wall lacerations may induce a hemo/pneumothorax.

Other considerations include the amount of irrigation and the temperature of the irrigant. In a study comparing different amounts of irrigation (250 cm^3, 500 cm^3, and 1000 cm^3), the incidence of infection was related inversely to the amount of irrigation; that is, the greater the irrigation, the lower was the incidence of infection.[30] A simple rule of thumb is to use 50 mL to 100 mL of irrigant per centimeter of laceration.[31] The more contaminated the wound, the greater the amount of irrigant required for proper wound preparation. Less irrigation may be acceptable with noncontaminated wounds in well-vascularized areas such as the face. Hollander and colleagues[32] found irrigation did not make a difference in clean, noncontaminated facial and scalp lacerations. When considering temperature of the irrigant, a single-blind, cross-over trial of irrigation of simple linear wounds demonstrated that warmed saline was more comfortable and soothing than room-temperature saline.[33]

Table 3
Agents for procedural sedation

Medication	Recommended Dose	Route of Administration
Fentanyl	1–3 μg/kg	Intravenous
Midazolam	0.02–0.1 mg/kg (adult) 0.05–0.15 mg/kg (child)	Intravenous
	0.05–0.15 mg/kg	Intramuscular
	0.5–0.75 mg/kg	Oral
Ketamine	1–2 mg/kg	Intravenous
	4–5 mg/kg	Intramuscular
Propofol	1 mg/kg	Intravenous
Etomidate	0.1–0.2 mg/kg	Intravenous

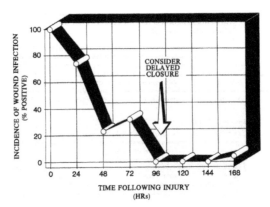

Fig. 1. This graph illustrates the best time for delayed wound closure from initial time of wounding. The incidence of infection is greatly reduced by 96 hours. (*From* Trott A. Decisions before closure–timing, debridement, consultation. In: Wounds and lacerations emergency care and closure. St. Louis (MO): Mosby; 1997. p. 119; with permission.)

If saline is not available for irrigation, tap water may be a good alternative. Several studies have shown tap water to be an effective irrigant without increasing rates of infection or growth of unusual organisms.[34–36] On the other hand, detergents, hydrogen peroxide, and concentrated povidone-iodine should be avoided in wound irrigation because these agents are toxic to tissues.[26,29] If detergent must be used (eg, to remove grease), it should be followed by copious irrigation.

Débridement should be reserved for wounds in which nonviable tissue creates a nidus for infection.[26,37] Necrotic tissue also obstructs re-epithelialization and wound contraction.[38] Therefore, all crushed or devitalized tissue should be debrided.

Hair should not be shaved during wound preparation. Bacteria reside in hair follicles, and shaving has been noted to increase wound infection.[26,39] Instead, clippers or scissors should be used to reduce damage to hair follicles.

Caps and masks have not been shown to make a difference in infection rates. Recently a prospective, randomized, multicenter trial evaluating the use of sterile versus nonsterile gloves in laceration repair showed no difference in the two groups in the final outcome of rate of infection as reported by patients on a questionnaire at the time of suture removal. Another randomized study has reproduced these results.[40] Sterile gloves fit better than nonsterile gloves, however, and result in better control of instruments and sutures. Sterile gloves continue to be used in most laceration repair.

Types of Wound Closure

There are three types of wound closure: primary, secondary, and delayed. Primary closure is closure of the wound before formation of granulation tissue. All "clean" wounds can be closed primarily except puncture wounds that cannot be irrigated adequately. Contaminated wounds, noncosmetic animal bites, abscess cavities, and wounds presenting after a delay should be irrigated, hemorrhage controlled, and debrided. Delayed primary closure can be performed after 3 to 5 days to allow the patient's defense system to decrease the bacterial load. Bacterial load will be at its lowest approximately 96 hours after the time of initial impact (**Fig. 1**). Secondary closure is healing by granulation tissue. This type of closure is suited for partial-thickness avulsions (ie, fingertip injuries), contaminated small wounds (ie, puncture wounds, stab wounds), and infected wounds.

Table 4	
Factors contributing to scar visibility	
Factors Associated with Scarring	**Methods to Minimize Scarring**
Direction of wound perpendicular to lines of static and dynamic tension	Layered closure; proper direction in elective incisions of wounds
Infection requiring removal of sutures and healing by secondary intention	Proper wound preparation; irrigation, and use of delayed closure in contaminated wounds
Wide scar secondary to tension	Layered closure, proper splinting, and elevation
Suture marks	Remove all percutaneous sutures within 7 days
Uneven wound edges	Careful, even approximation of wound superficial layer to prevent differential swelling of edges
Inversion of wound edges	Proper placement of simple sutures or use of horizontal mattress sutures
Tattooing secondary to retained dirt or foreign body	Proper wound preparation and débridement
Tissue necrosis	Use of corner sutures on flaps, splinting, and elevation of wounds with marginal circulation or venous return; excision of nonviable wound edges before closure
Compromised healing secondary to hematoma	Use of properly conforming dressing and splints
Hyperpigmentation of scar or abraded skin	Use of sun block with a sun protection factor $\geq$ 15 for 6 months
Superimposition of blood clots between healing wound edges	Proper hemostasis and closure; proper application of compressive dressings
Failure to align anatomic structures (eg, vermilion border) properly	Meticulous closure and alignment; use of regional blocks

Adapted from Markovchick V. Suture materials and mechanical after care. Emerg Med Clin North Am 1992;10:676.

Techniques of Wound Closure

The balance between function and cosmesis is a major consideration in selecting the technique for wound closure. When the goal is to obtain the best function, the laceration should be closed in a single layer with the least amount of sutures. When cosmesis is most important, a multiple-layer closure should be used.[41] Intradermal sutures when placed in areas of high static and dynamic wound tension improve cosmesis by facilitating the placement of surface sutures. Singer and colleagues[42] evaluated determinants of poor outcome after laceration repair. In their evaluation the type of closure and the use of deep sutures had no effect on cosmesis or infection rates, but the wounds included in the study were small, with mean length of 2.2 ± 1.9 cm and mean width of 3.5 ± 3.8 mm. **Table 4** lists the factors to consider when cosmesis is of utmost importance.

Stellate wounds that change directions or have multiple components are best closed with simple interrupted sutures. This type of suture would not be ideal for a wound with increased tension caused by swelling. For a wound under increased tension, such as over joints, horizontal mattress sutures can be used in a single-layer closure because they are naturally everting, hemostatic, and do not cut through skin edges if tension increases from movement or swelling. This type of closure is not used when the primary goal is cosmesis. Running sutures can be used in wounds under minimal tension or as the surface sutures in a layered closure.

Some lacerations need further manipulation by the clinician in preparation for closure. In gaping wounds, skin tension can be reduced by undermining the wound. Undermining is the procedure by which the dermis and superficial fascia are released from deeper attachments, allowing wound edges to be brought together with less force. Undermining should be performed to a distance from the wound edge that approximates the extent of gaping of the wound edges.[43]

Lacerations that are irregular in configuration and depth may require use of a mix of different techniques for closure. Triangular and circular lacerations can be converted into elliptical lacerations for better closure.

Materials

Various options are available for wound closure including sutures, staples, tissue adhesives, and adhesive tapes. Although each modality has its place in wound management, it is important to assess wound characteristics carefully to make the best choice in material.

Sutures

When selecting sutures the clinician must make two further decisions: absorbable versus nonabsorbable sutures and needle size. Absorbable sutures typically are used to close structures deeper than the epidermis. The synthetic absorbable sutures are less reactive and maintain greater tensile strength than the natural sources. The epidermis then is closed with nonabsorbable sutures such as nylon or polypropylene. The advantage of sutures over adhesives for this surface closure is that sutures can be used to ensure the opposed wound edges are even. These nonabsorbable sutures are relatively nonreactive and retain tensile strength for longer than 60 days.[26,41]

Karounis and colleagues compared cosmetic outcomes in traumatic pediatric lacerations closed with absorbable plain gut versus nonabsorbable nylon sutures. There was no difference between the groups in rates of deshiscence or infection. Plain gut also provided slightly better cosmesis.[44] When Luck and colleagues compared the use of absorbable and nonabsorbable sutures for closure of pediatric facial lacerations there were no significant differences in complication rates or parental satisfaction.[45] An additional benefit of using absorbable sutures is avoidance of the added distress to the patient of suture removal. A study in the dermatology literature, suggests that this is a viable option in adults as well.[46]

Needle size depends on the location of the wound (**Table 5**). Typically, the epidermis is closed with 6.0 sutures on the face and 4.0 or 5.0 sutures on the extremities. Deep stitches typically are placed with 4.0 or 5.0 sutures.

Staples

Staples are a cosmetically acceptable alternative to sutures for the closure of scalp lacerations[47] and also are used for closure of linear perpendicular lacerations of the scalp, trunk, or extremities. Care must be taken to avoid uneven or overlapping wound edges when placing staples. Studies comparing staples and sutures have shown that staples provide more rapid wound repair[47–49] and have a lower rate of reactivity and infection.[49] The disadvantages of staples are the inability to provide a meticulous closure and the more painful process of removal.[48]

Table 5
Guidelines for suture material dependent on body region

Body Region	Suture Material (Skin)	Suture Material (Deep)	Special Closure and Dressing	Suture Removal
Scalp	3-0 or 4-0 NA	4-0 SA	Interrupted in galea; single, tight layer for scalp	7–12 d
Pinna (ear)	6-0 NA	5-0 SA	Interrupted SA sutures for perichondrium; stint dressing	4–6 d
Eyebrow	6-0 NA	4-0 or 5-0 SA	Layered closure	4–5 d
Eyelid	6-0 NA	None	Single-layer horizontal mattress	4–5 d
Lip	6-0 NA	4-0 silk or SA (mucosa); 5-0 SA (subcutaneous, muscle)	Three-layered closure for through and through lacerations	4–6 d
Oral cavity	None	4-0 SA	Layered closure if muscularis of tongue involved	7–8 d or allow to dissolve
Face	6-0 NA	4-0 or 5-0 SA	Layered closure for full-thickness lacerations	4–6 d
Neck	5-0 NA	4-0 SA (subcutaneous)	Two-layered closure gives best cosmetic result	4–6 d
Trunk	4-0 or 5-0 NA	4-0 SA (subcutaneous, fat)	Single or layered closure	7–12 d
Extremity	4-0 or 5-0 NA	3-0 or 4-0 SA (subcutaneous, fat, muscle)	Splint if wound is over a joint	7–14 d
Hands and feet	4-0 or 5-0 NA	None	Only close skin; use horizontal mattress sutures if there is much tension on wound edges; splint if wound over joint	7–12 d
Nailbed	5-0 SA	None	Replace nail under cuticle	Allow to dissolve

Abbreviations: NA, nonabsorbable suture (eg, nylon, polypropylene); SA, synthetic absorbable suture.
Data from Markovchick V. Soft tissue injury and wound repair. In: Reisdorff EJ, Roberts MR, Wiegenstein JG, editors. Pediatric emergency medicine. Philadelphia: W.B. Saunders; 1993. p. 899–908; and Trott A. Special anatomic sites. In: Wounds and lacerations emergency care and closure. St. Louis (MO): Mosby; 1997. p. 179.

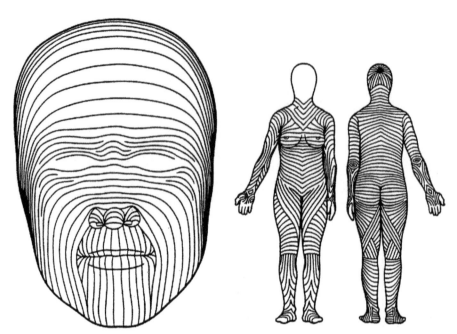

Fig. 2. Direction of lines of skin tension. (*From* Marx J, Hockberger R, Well R, et al, editors. Rosen's emergency medicine: concepts and clinical practice. 5th edition. Philadelphia: Mosby; 2002. p. 738–9; with permission.)

Tissue Adhesives

The cyanoacrylate adhesives were developed in 1945 to be applied topically to the epidermis, thus bridging the wound edges. Care must be taken to avoid getting any adhesive between cut wound edges. Although considered a relatively painless method of wound closure, the chemical reaction of polymerization when tissue adhesives are applied produces heat that can cause some discomfort.[31] Wound closure using this method is less painful and faster than closure with sutures. Tissue adhesive is an effective method of closing appropriately selected wounds. Use of tissue adhesives should be limited to linear lacerations less than 4 cm in length[50] in wounds devoid of significant tension or repetitive movement. If tissue adhesive is used to close the skin in an area of high tension, subcutaneous or subcuticular sutures are required to relieve this tension.

One of the largest studies comparing tissue adhesives with sutures was the manufacturer-sponsored study for the approval of 2-octylcyanoacrylate by the Food and Drug Administration. This study found that tissue adhesives had performance comparable to sutures in short-term infection rate, wound dehiscence, and 3-month cosmetic outcome.[26,51] Other studies have shown similar results.[52,53] When used for wound repair in athletes allowed to return to play immediately, tissue adhesive was found to retain its strength, durability, and skin apposition.[54]

Wounds parallel to Langer's lines of skin tension tend to have a better outcome than those running against these physiologic lines (**Fig. 2**). Simon[55] evaluated facial lacerations closed with tissue adhesives or sutures, specifically studying laceration relationship to lines of skin tension. All wounds greater than 5 mm in length underwent placement of subcutaneous sutures. Then patients were assigned randomly to tissue adhesives or sutures for skin closure. He noted that cosmetic outcome of facial lacerations repaired by tissue adhesives was less affected by the initial orientation of the wound. The author's concluded that tissue adhesives can be used to close facial lacerations regardless of the orientation of the wound.[55] Several techniques are available for the removal of these tissue adhesives. Bathing accelerates removal, as does the application of antibiotic ointment or petroleum jelly. If more rapid removal is necessary, acetone can be used.

Adhesive Tapes

Studies have shown adhesive tapes to be equal to staples in cosmesis and to pose less risk of infection than either staples or sutures.[56] Lacerations evaluated in this study were facial lacerations less than 2.5 cm in length and less than 12 hours old. Cosmetic outcomes were evaluated at 2 months, which may not correlate with long-term outcome.

Adhesive tapes can be applied in many different patterns, but a parallel, non-overlapping pattern with complete coating of the skin surface with Liquid adhesive has the highest degree of adherence.[57] At 10 days these wounds have tensile strength equal or superior to that of wounds closed with sutures.[57]

Special Situations in Wound Management

Scalp

A scalp wound requires palpation and exploration for the evaluation of a possible skull fracture. After proper exploration, the wound edges should be approximated tightly with sutures or staples to prevent hematoma formation. The double staple gun technique is a useful trick for use in pediatric lacerations requiring two staples. This technique involves two physicians holding a staple gun perpendicular to the laceration and firing the staple gun in unison. Placing the staples at the same time is less painful and decreases the emotional trauma for the patient.[58]

Scalp lacerations 3 to 10 cm in length also can be closed using the patient's own hair. Hair strands need to be at least 3 cm in length. Strands from each side of the wound are twisted together to approximate the wound edges. The intertwined strands then are secured in place using a drop of tissue adhesive. This procedure is quick and cost effective as well as less painful for the patient.[58]

Pinna

Anesthesia of the pinna is obtained with a field block. After repair, a pressure dressing must be applied to prevent formation of a hematoma between the skin and the perichondrium. A hematoma in this site is painful and may compromise the blood supply to the cartilage. The dressing is left in place for 24 to 48 hours.

The wound needs to be inspected for any cartilaginous involvement. These lacerations are closed by apposing the skin overlying the laceration in the cartilage. In a through-and-through laceration, the anterior and posterior portions of the wound are closed separately. If possible, one should avoid placing sutures through the cartilage. If the skin cannot be brought over the cartilage without tension, conservative débridement must be performed. No more than 5 mm of cartilage should be debrided. More than that will deform the cartilaginous skeleton.[59]

Eyebrow

Excision of tissue is to be avoided. When débridement is necessary, it should be performed in a parallel direction of the hair follicle. Eyebrows should never be removed, because doing so can lead to abnormal growth. The eyebrow provides a useful guide for approximation of wound edges.

Eyelid

Eyelid lacerations require an examination for possible globe penetration. If the laceration is through the tarsal plate or involves the lacrimal apparatus, an ophthalmology consultation is advised. If simple sutures result in inversion or overlapping of wound edges, horizontal mattress sutures should be used.

Lip

Through-and-through lip lacerations require layered closure from the inside out. Suturing the oral mucosa first minimizes contamination of the wound from saliva. After the mucosa is closed with absorbable suture, the closure is checked by irrigating the wound and evaluating for leaks into the oral cavity. Subsequently the muscle layer is closed with 4.0 or 5.0 absorbable suture. Not closing the muscle layer can lead to a depression of the scar as the muscle fibers retract. In closing the outer aspect of the lip, priority is given to approximating the vermilion border with the first stitch or "stay" suture placed at this site. If part of the vermillion is missing with the laceration, a full-thickness wedge of lip tissue can be removed. This technique will produce a single linear scar with an intact vermilion, which is preferable to an irregular vermillion margin. Up to one third of the lip can be lost without appreciable distortion in the symmetry of the lip.[60] Because of the importance of the approximation of the vermilion border, regional anesthesia (infraorbital or mental nerve block) should be considered.

Oral cavity and mucous membranes

Lacerations of the buccal mucosa and gingiva generally heal without repair, but wounds that are longer than 2 cm, gaping, or continuing to bleed should be closed tightly with absorbable 4.0 or 5.0 suture. Likewise, the indications for repair of tongue lacerations are uncontrollable hemorrhage, airway compromise, the presence of a significant segment of severed tongue, or a gaping laceration. Tongue sutures should be placed wide and deep. These sutures should be tied loosely to allow room for swelling. Placing an instrument such as a closed hemostat between the suture and the tongue prevents overtying the knot.[60] All three layers (inferior mucosa, muscle, and superior mucosa) of a tongue laceration can be closed with one stitch or with two stitches including half of the thickness of the tongue in each stitch. If the wound involves the posterior pharynx, a lateral soft tissue radiograph may be of benefit in determining the extent of the wound. Air dissecting along fascial planes is indicative of deep space involvement.

Face

With cheek lacerations, there is potential for injury to the parotid gland and to the seventh cranial nerve. Discharge of clear fluid from the wound indicates parotid gland or Stensen's duct involvement. Involvement of these structures is an indication for consultation. Facial wounds should not undergo radical débridement. Because of the excellent blood supply to the head and neck, tissue can survive in this region on small pedicles.[60]

Extremities

Lacerations over joints need to be evaluated for involvement of the joint capsule. Sterile saline can be injected into the joint to assess for a defect in the joint capsule.

Extravasation is better appreciated by adding a few drops of methylene blue to the saline. Small defects in the capsule can be detected by the use of fluorescein. A drop of fluorescein is placed into 50 mL of saline and injected into the joint. The joint then is wrapped for 10 minutes. Once the wrap is removed, extravasation can be detected with a Wood's lamp.[61]

Wounds over joints or under increased tension require suturing with interrupted horizontal mattress sutures and splinting for at least 1 to 2 weeks.

Hands

Conservative treatment with serial nonadherent dressings is advocated for pulp defects less than 1 cm^2 in adults and proportionately smaller in children with minimal or no bone exposure.[62] Lacerations less than 2 cm also may be treated conservatively without suturing. Quinn and colleagues[63] evaluated hand lacerations less than 2 cm long without associated tendon, joint, bone, or nerve injury. They randomly assigned patients to conservative management or suturing. Two independent physicians blinded to treatment assessed the end points. Cosmetic appearance at 3 months did not differ between the two groups. The mean time to treatment, however, was longer in the suture group than in the conservative group (19 minutes vs 5 minutes). Time to resume normal activities was reported as the same in both groups.[63,64]

Many factors must be considered when deciding between replantation or amputation of a distal digit injury. In a study from Japan, replantation provided better functional outcomes, better appearance, and higher patient satisfaction with minimal pain. The other disadvantage of amputation is the potential for a painful stump. On the other hand, amputation provides a shorter recovery period and faster return to work.[65]

Nail bed

The nail bed is damaged in 15% to 24% of fingertip injuries in children.[62] Simple lacerations through the sterile matrix can be repaired with 6.0 or 7.0 absorbable suture[62] or with the use of 2-otylcyanoacrylate. Both methods provide similar cosmetic and functional results.[66] If the nail plate has been removed, it should be replaced to maintain adequate space between the germinal matrix and the proximal nail fold. A small hole can be placed in the nail bed to allow for drainage. The nail plate then is secured with a 5.0 nylon suture through the hyponychium or with a horizontal mattress suture through the proximal nail fold. If a distal hyponychium suture is used, it can be left in place for 7 to 10 days. The nail plate also has been replaced using tissue adhesives[67,68] and chloramphenicol.[69] With chloramphenicol, a small amount of ointment is applied to the deep surface of the nail plate, and then the nail plate is slipped under the eponychial fold into position. The ointment forms an adhesive layer between the nail plate and the nail bed. The finger then is dressed, and the dressing is left in place for 1 week. The nail plate works itself loose on its own, usually when that occurs the nail bed is well healed and the new nail is growing from below. If the nail plate is not available, a piece of reinforced silicone sheeting or nonadherent gauze can be used instead.

For subungal hematomas there is no difference between nail bed removal with repair of the nail bed laceration and drainage of the hematoma without nail removal. The results of one study recommended conservative management of subungal hematoma regardless of size when the nail plate is still adherent to the bed and not displaced out of the nail folds. Roser and Gellman[70] compared nail trephinization and nail bed repair for subungal hematoma in children. Inclusion criteria for the study were an intact nail and nail margin with subungal hematoma and no previous nail

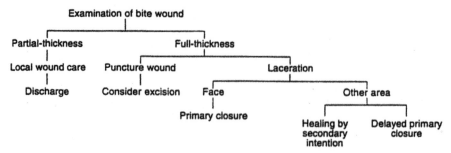

Fig. 3. Algorithm for the care of bite wounds. (*From* Markovchick V. Wound management. In: Markovchick V, Pons P, editors. Emergency medicine secrets. Philadelphia: Mosby Elsevier; 2006. p. 666; with permission.)

abnormality. These authors found no difference in outcome for the two groups regardless of hematoma size, presence of fracture, age, or injury mechanism.

About 50% of nail bed injuries have an associated distal phalangeal fracture.[70] Although these injuries usually can be considered open fractures, antibiotics are not indicated for this type of wound.

Bites

Five percent of traumatic wounds evaluated in the ED result from mammalian bites, most commonly dog bites. Infection rates are highest for puncture wounds caused by cat bites, ranging from 29% to 50%.[71] Chen and colleagues[72] studied primary closure of wounds caused by mammalian bites (dogs, cats, humans) and found the overall infection rate to be 6%. There was no difference between the incidence of infection in lacerations of the head and the upper extremities. This infection rate may be acceptable when closure is necessary and cosmesis is the main concern. **Fig. 3** gives a suggested algorithm to be used for the care of bite wounds.

Gunshot wounds

The increased damage associated with high-velocity injuries is secondary to the dissipation of kinetic energy. Also, behind the bullet there is a sucking action that deposits clothing or dirt in the wound. Wounds caused by bullets should be debrided, irrigated, and left open to be repaired with delayed primary closure or by secondary closure.

ANTIBIOTICS IN WOUND CARE

One of the continuing controversies in wound management is the use of prophylactic antibiotics. Studies looking at antibiotics in wound care have varied in definitions of infection and in protocols for outpatient wound surveillance. These studies also have been limited by the low number of subjects.

In 1961 Burke[73] looked at the effective period for preventive antibiotics in contaminated wounds. He noted this period to be from the time bacteria gained access to the wound to 2 to 3 hours after the initial inoculation. This finding suggests a golden period for administration of antibiotics of 3 hours to limit bacterial proliferation. When evaluating clinical studies, this estimate seems to be conservative.

Several studies have failed to show a benefit for prophylactic antibiotics in simple lacerations.[4,26,74–76] After performing a meta-analysis of randomized trials of prophylactic antibiotics for simple nonbite wounds, Cummings and Del Beccaro[77] concluded that there is no evidence that this practice offers protection against infection.

Whittaker and colleagues[78] performed a prospective randomized, placebo-controlled, double-blinded study in adults looking at the use of antibiotics in clean, incised hand injuries including trauma to the skin, tendon, and nerve. Wound infection was defined as frank purulence, greater erythema than expected, or wound dehiscence. Infection also included a wound problem with a pathogenic bacterial growth on microbiologic swab results. Mild erythema or serous discharge without bacterial growth on swabs was described as a wound problem. Infection rates were 15% for placebo, 13% for intravenous flucloxacillin (a narrow-spectrum beta-lactam antibiotic), and 4% for the combination of intravenous antibiotic followed by an oral regimen. These differences were not statistically significant.[78] It is unclear, however, if antibiotics would benefit specific subgroups of patients who have characteristics placing them at a higher risk of infection (ie, diabetes mellitus). Antibiotics are indicated in patients prone to bacterial endocarditis, those who have an orthopedic prosthesis, and those who have lymphedema.

Because oral injuries are assumed to be contaminated with micro-organisms, it has been suggested that these wounds should be supported with prophylactic antibiotics. Clinical evidence for the use of antibiotics in this setting is lacking, however. The use of antibiotics for an oral wound may be warranted in heavily contaminated wounds where débridement is not optimal; wounds in which débridement is delayed for more than 24 hours; wounds associated with open reduction of jaw fractures; wounds in patients who have compromised defense systems; and wounds caused by human or animal bites.[60]

Evidence supports the use of antibiotics in hand injuries involving fractures, contaminated wounds, crush injuries, animal bites, and human bites.[78] Zubowicz and Gravier[79] found mechanical wound care by itself to be insufficient therapy for human bites of the hand. In their study, oral and intravenous antibiotics were equivalent for prophylaxis.

Further evaluation of hand injuries involving fractures suggest that not all hand fractures associated with wounds warrant antibiotics. A study looking at the prophylactic use of flucloxacillin in the treatment of open fractures of the distal phalanx showed that the antibiotics did not confer any benefit over thorough wound preparation and careful soft tissue repair.[80]

In dog bite wounds, débridement is more effective than prophylactic antibiotics in reducing infection. One study evaluating care of dog bites showed a 68% rate of infection in wounds without débridement, compared with an infection rate of 2% in the débridement group.[81] Wounds that could not be irrigated thoroughly, such as puncture wounds, had an infection rate twice that of wounds that could be irrigated thoroughly.[81] Therefore, high-risk wounds such as those on the hand or puncture wounds benefit from prophylactic antibiotics. Antibiotics are not required in low-risk wounds, such as deep wounds that can be adequately irrigated or in wounds of the face or scalp.

In conclusion, antibiotics are not beneficial in clean wounds even when these wounds involve the hand. In general, antibiotics are recommended for contaminated wounds or wounds that cannot be adequately debrided or irrigated. Also antibiotics need to be considered in patients who are more prone to infection including diabetics. Each wound needs to be considered individually, and the patient should have good follow-up, especially when the clinician decides not to provide antibiotics in potentially high-risk wounds.

COSMESIS

Although all wounds heal with a scar, the final appearance of this scar is influenced by patient factors, wound factors, and technical factors. Important patient factors include comorbid conditions, age, ethnicity, skin type, medications, and hereditary predisposition.[82] Wound factors include the nature of the wound (elective vs traumatic), location and orientation of the wound, vascularity of the tissues, elasticity and tension of soft tissues, and degree of contamination. Technical factors include the handling of tissues, débridement, sutures used, and method of wound repair. Avoiding rough tissue handling and the use of crushing instruments is important in preventing tissue ischemia, which leads to necrosis and poor scarring.

Wounds continue to remodel over 3 to 12 months. During that time period the scar may widen. Therefore, the long-term cosmetic outcome of the wound may not correlate with the short-term outcome.[26]

Factors associated with patient-rated cosmesis scores may differ from those associated with doctor-rated cosmesis scores. Lowe and colleagues[83] found cosmetic outcome was the most important aspect of wound care for 33% of patients who had facial wounds and 17% of all patients who had lacerations. Patients in Lowe's study judged scar appearance using a 10-point numerical rating scale 14 days after repair and 3 months after repair. The site of laceration was the most significant factor related to satisfactory patient-rated cosmesis. Lacerations on the torso, leg, or foot received the lowest cosmesis scores. Another factor associated with poor cosmetic outcomes was increased time from injury to repair. Seniority of the practitioner performing the repair was not a significant factor in patient-rated cosmesis.

AFTERCARE INSTRUCTIONS

If possible wounds should be covered with a nonadherent dressing for 24 to 48 hours. This period allows enough epithelialization to protect the wound from contamination.[28] Compression dressings should be applied to wounds with potential for hematoma formation. This dressing is left in place for 24 to 48 hours. After this time period, dressings should be removed, and wounds should be cleaned three to four times a day to minimize coagulum between wound edges. Thereafter, patients should be advised to administer a sun-blocking agent with a sun protective factor of 15 to the wound to prevent hyperpigmentation from exposure to sunlight. This process should be continued for 6 months.

Tissue adhesives do not require removal and will slough off over 5 to 10 days with wound epithelialization. Sutures and staples require removal on an average of 7 days after placement. Facial sutures can be removed in 3 to 5 days to avoid formation of sinus tracts. Sutures over joints or areas with a lot of movement should stay in for 10 to 14 days. Also lacerations overlying joint surfaces should be splinted in position of function for up to 10 days.

FUTURE OF WOUND CARE
Anesthesia with Nitrous Oxide

Bar-Meir and colleagues[84] evaluated the administration of nitrous oxide for repair of facial lacerations by plastic surgeons in the ED. The appealing aspects of this drug are its fast onset and rapid recovery characteristics, which make it an ideal drug for short procedures. It provides analgesia, anxiolysis, amnesia, and euphoria while having minimal cardiovascular and respiratory effects. The American Society of Anesthesiologists considers 50% nitrous oxide in oxygen as minimal sedation. Because administration of nitrous oxide requires a mask, there may be some limitations to its use. These investigators used a nasal mask for the administration of the drug, leaving the mouth uncovered. The mask could be removed immediately in case of emesis. The only lacerations covered by the mask were those on the nose. For nasal lacerations, the gas was administered first, followed by infiltration of local anesthetic while the patient was still under the influence of the gas. Also, because 50% nitrous oxide allows patients to maintain normal airway reflexes, fasting was not required before anesthesia. The authors of this study concluded that nitrous oxide could be safely administered in the ED.[84]

Botulinum Toxin

One group of investigators looked at the use of botulinum toxin in the repair of facial wounds. The study included 31 patients who had traumatic forehead lacerations or were undergoing elective excision of forehead masses. Patients were assigned randomly to injection of either botulinum toxin or placebo into the musculature in a diameter of approximately 1 to 3 cm around wound edges within 24 hours of wound closure. Immobilizing the wounds with the toxin enhanced healing and led to a superior cosmetic appearance at 6 months.[85] Further studies need to evaluate the use of chemoimmobilization in other types of lacerations in multiple different sites. Although this therapy may be a part of the future of wound management, its use in the ED may be limited by its cost.

Porcine Small Intestinal Mucosa

Kragh and colleagues[86] reported better results in supination torque, appearance, and satisfaction when muscle was repaired with suture than with nonoperative management. Porcine SIS is a collagenous biomaterial that induces site-specific remodeling of various connective tissues. This product can act as a collagen scaffold allowing ingrowth of host tissue appropriate to the location of implantation. This product was tested on full-thickness muscle belly lacerations in rabbits. The study suggested that SIS, when added to a suture repair of muscle, may improve final outcomes and function.[87] The healed tissue after repair with SIS resembled normal muscle in morphology and function more closely than did nonsutured tissue, sutured tissue without use of SIS, or nonsutured tissue with use of SIS. At this time it is unclear if this product will be available for ED management of muscle wounds.

Hyaluronidase Injections

Wounds from human bites typically are allowed to repair by secondary intention or undergo delayed closure. A new method described in the literature is the use of hyaluronidase injections around the wound site allowing immediate closure of wounds that otherwise might be considered for delayed closure. This product enzymatically breaks up the intercellular cement substance. When combined with external pressure in wounds, there is a diffusion of fluid exudates into the open wound and away from the wound margins. This process results in a soft, flattened wound facilitating closure without tension.[88] This process eliminates wound edema in minutes instead of days.

The use of hyaluronidase has been evaluated in the treatment of bite wounds in the orofacial area. In the cases reviewed, 2 to 3 mL of hyaluronidase were injected into the wound margins, with pressure being held for at least 10 minutes. All wounds healed uneventfully between 17 days and 1 month after injury. Hyaluronidase is not available currently for wounds treated in the ED.

SUMMARY

To treat wounds properly, the emergency physician needs knowledge of basic wound physiology along with host and wound factors affecting healing. Although many options are available for wound closure, the choice of closure needs to be appropriate for the wound. Wound and host factors affect the type of closure that is best for different types of wounds. The ultimate goal is to obtain the ideal functional and cosmetic result without complications.

REFERENCES

1. National Hospital Ambulatory Medical Care Survey. Emergency department summary. Advance data from vital and health statistics; no. 293. National centre for health statistics 1996. Available at: http://www.cdc.gov/nchs/data/ad/ad293.pdf. Accessed March 2007.
2. Trott A. Surface injury and wound healing. In: Wounds and lacerations emergency care and closure. St. Louis (MO): Mosby; 1991. p. 12–23.
3. Cruse PJE, Foord R. A five-year prospective study of 23,649 surgical wounds. Arch Surg 1973;107:206–9.
4. Stamou SC, Maltezou HC, Psaltopoulou T, et al. Wound infections after minor limb lacerations: risk factors and the role of antimicrobial agents. J Trauma 1999;46(6): 1078–81.
5. Pulaski EJ, Meleney FL, Spacth WL. Bacterial flora of acute traumatic wounds. Surg Gynecol Obstet 1941;72:982–8.
6. Robson MC, Duke WF, Krizek TJ, et al. Rapid bacterial screening in the treatment of civilian wounds. J Surg Res 1973;14:426–30.
7. Berk WA, Osbourne DD, Taylor DD. Evaluation of the 'golden period' for wound repair: 204 cases from a third world emergency department. Ann Emerg Med 1988;17(5):496–500.
8. Berk WA, Welch RD, Bock BF. Controversial issues in clinical management of the simple wound. Ann Emerg Med 1992;21(1):72–80.
9. Pascual FB, McGinley EL, Zanardi LR, et al. Tetanus surveillance–United States, 1998-2000. MMWR Morb Mortal Wkly Rep 2003;52(SS03):1–8.
10. Centers for Disease Control. Morbidity and mortality weekly report. Available at: http://www.cdc.gov/mmwr/preview/mmwrhtml. Accessed March 2007.
11. Hollander JE, Singer AJ, Valentine SM, et al. Risk factors for infection in patients with traumatic lacerations. Acad Emerg Med 2001;8:716–20.
12. Chisholm CD. Wound evaluation and cleansing. Emerg Med Clin North Am 1992; 10(4):665–72.
13. Lammers RL, Magill T. Detection and management of foreign bodies in soft tissue. Emerg Med Clin North Am 1992;10(40):767–80.
14. Anderson MA, Newmeyer WL, Kilgore ES. Diagnosis and treatment of retained foreign bodies in the hand. Am J Surg 1982;144:63–7.
15. Singer AJ, Stark MJ. Pretreatment of lacerations with lidocaine, epinephrine, and tetracaine at triage: a randomized double-blind trial. Acad Emerg Med 2000;7(7):751–6.
16. Kelly AM, Cohen M, Richards D. Minimizing the pain of local infiltration anesthesia for wounds by injection into the wound edges. J Emerg Med 1994;12:593–5.
17. Bartfield JM, Sokaris SJ, Raccio-Robak N. Local anesthesia for lacerations: pain of infiltration inside vs. outside the wound. Acad Emerg Med 1998;5:100–4.
18. Edlich RF, Rodeheaver GT, Morgan RF, et al. Principles of emergency wound management. Ann Emerg Med 1988;17:1284–302.
19. Bartfield JM, Gennis P, Barbera J, et al. Buffered versus plain lidocaine as a local anesthetic for simple laceration repair. Ann Emerg Med 1990;19(12):1387–9.
20. Brogan GX, Jr., Giarrusso E, Hollander JE, et al. Comparison of plain, warmed, and buffered lidocaine for anesthesia of traumatic wounds. Ann Emerg Med 1995;26(2):121–5.
21. Bartfield JM, Lee FS, Raccio-Robak N, et al. Topical tetracaine attenuates the pain of infiltration of buffered lidocaine. Acad Emerg Med 1996;3:1001–5.

22. Sacchetti A, Senula G, Strickland J, et al. Procedural sedation in the community emergency department: initial results of the ProSCED registry. Acad Emerg Med 2007;14:41–6.
23. Sinha M, Christopher NC, Fenn R, et al. Evaluation of nonpharmacologic methods of pain and anxiety management for laceration repair in the pediatric emergency department. Pediatrics 2006;117(4):1162–8.
24. Hamer ML, Martin CR, Krizek TJ, et al. Quantitative bacterial analysis of comparative wound irrigations. Ann Surg 1975;181(6):819–22.
25. Dire DJ, Welsh AP. A comparison of wound irrigation solutions used in the emergency department. Ann Emerg Med 1990;19:704–8.
26. Hollander JE, Singer AJ. Laceration management. Ann Emerg Med 1999;34(3): 356–67.
27. Stevenson TR, Thacker JG, Rodeheaver GT, et al. Cleansing the traumatic wound by high pressure syringe irrigation. JACEP 1976;5(1):17–21.
28. Singer AJ, Hollander JE, Quinn JV. Evaluation and management of traumatic lacerations. N Engl J Med 1997;337(16):1142–8.
29. Dulecki M, Pieper B. Irrigating simple acute traumatic wounds: a review of the current literature. J Emerg Nurs 2005;31(2):156–60.
30. Peterson LW. Prophylaxis of wound infection. Arch Surg 1945;50(4):177–83.
31. Knapp JF. Updates in wound management for the pediatrician. Pediatr Clin North Am 1999;46(6):1201–13.
32. Hollander JE, Richman PB, Werblud M, et al. Irrigation in facial and scalp lacerations: does it alter outcome? Ann Emerg Med 1998;31(1):73–7.
33. Ernst AA, Gershoff L, Miller P, et al. Warmed versus room temperature saline for laceration irrigation: a randomized clinical trial. South Med J 2003;96(5):436–9.
34. Moscati RM, Reardon RF, Lerner EB, et al. Wound irrigation with tap water. Acad Emerg Med 1998;5:1076–80.
35. Moscati R, Mayrose J, Fincher L, et al. Comparison of normal saline with tap water for wound irrigation. Am J Emerg Med 1998;16:379–81.
36. Bansal BC, Wiebe RA, Perkins SD, et al. Tap water for irrigation of lacerations. Am J Emerg Med 2002;20:469–72.
37. Haury B, Rodeheaver G, Vensko J, et al. Debridement: an essential component of traumatic wound care. Am J Surg 1978;135(2):238–42.
38. Schultz GS, Sibbald RG, Falanga V, et al. Wound bed preparation: a systematic approach to wound management. Wound Repair Regen 2003;11:1–28.
39. Seropian R, Reynolds BM. Wound infections after preoperative depilation versus razor preparation. Am J Surg 1971;121:251–4.
40. Perelman VS, Francis GJ, Rutledge T, et al. Sterile versus nonsterile gloves for repair of uncomplicated lacerations in the emergency department: a randomized controlled trial. Ann Emerg Med 2004;43:362–70.
41. Markovchick V. Suture materials and mechanical after care. Emerg Med Clin North Am 1992;10(4):673–89.
42. Singer AJ, Quinn JV, Thode HC Jr, et al. Determinants of poor outcome after laceration and surgical incision repair. Plast Reconstr Surg 2002;110(2):429–35.
43. Trott A. Basic laceration repair principles and techniques. In: Falk KH, editor. Wounds and lacerations emergency care and closure. St. Louis (MO): Mosby; 1997. p. 132–53.
44. Karounis H, Gouin S, Eisman H, et al. A randomized, controlled trial comparing long-term cosmetic outcomes of traumatic pediatric lacerations repaired with absorbable plain gut versus nonabsorbable nylon sutures. Acad Emerg Med 2004:11; 730–5.

45. Luck RP, Flood R, Eyal D, et al. Cosmetic outcomes of absorbable versus nonabsorbable sutures in pediatric facial lacerations. Pediatr Emerg Care 2008;24(3):137–42.

46. Rosenzweig LB, Abdelmalek M, Ho J, et al. Equal cosmetic outcomes with 5-0 poliglecaprone-25 versus 6-0 polypropylene for superficial closures. Dermatol Surg 2010;36(7):1126–9.

47. Khan A, Dayan PS, Miller S, et al. Cosmetic outcome of scalp wound closure with staples in the pediatric emergency department: a prospective, randomized trial. Pediatr Emerg Care 2002;18(3):171–3.

48. George TK, Simpson DC. Skin wound closure with staples in the accident and emergency department. J R Coll Surg Edinb 1985;30(1):54–6.

49. Kanegaye JT, Vance CW, Chan L, et al. Comparison of skin stapling devices and standard sutures for pediatric scalp lacerations: a randomized study of cost and time benefits. J Pediatr 1997;130:808–13.

50. Lo S, Aslam N. A review of tissue glue use in facial lacerations: potential problems with wound selection in accident and emergency. Eur J Emerg Med 2004;11(5):277–9.

51. Singer AJ, Quinn JV, Clark RE, et al. Closure of lacerations and incisions with octylcyanoacrylate: a multicenter randomized controlled trial. Surgery 2002;131: 270–6.

52. Quinn J, Wells G, Sutcliffe T, et al. A randomized trial comparing octylcyanoacrylate tissue adhesive and sutures in the management of lacerations. JAMA 1997;277(19): 1527–30.

53. Simon HK, McLario DJ, Bruns TB, et al. Long-term appearance of lacerations repaired using a tissue adhesive. Pediatrics 1997;99:193–5.

54. Perron AD, Garcia JA, Hays EP, et al. The efficacy of cyanoacrylate-derived surgical adhesive for use in the repair of lacerations during competitive athletics. Am J Emerg Med 2000;18(3):261–3.

55. Simon HK, Zempsky WT, Bruns TB, et al. Lacerations against Langer's lines: to glue or suture? J Emerg Med 1998;16(2):185–9.

56. Zempsky WT, Parrotti D, Grem C, et al. Randomized controlled comparison of cosmetic outcomes of simple facial lacerations closed with Steri strip skin closures or Dermabond tissue adhesive. Pediatr Emerg Care 2004;20(8):519–24.

57. Katz KH, Desciak EB, Maloney ME. The optimal application of surgical adhesive tape strips. Dermatol Surg 1999;25(9):686–8.

58. Lin M, Milan M. Managing scalp lacerations. ACEP News 2007;30.

59. Trott A. Special anatomic sites. In: Falk KH, editor. Wounds and lacerations emergency care and closure. St. Louis (MO): Mosby; 1997. p. 178–207.

60. Armstrong BD. Lacerations of the mouth. Emerg Med Clin North Am 2000;18(3): 471–80.

61. Zukin DD, Simon RR. Regional care. In: Emergency wound care principles and practice. Rockville (MD): Aspen Publishers, Inc; 1987. p. 77–109.

62. de Alwis W. Fingertip injuries. Emerg Med Australas 2006;18:229–37.

63. Quinn J, Cummings S, Callaham M, et al. Suturing versus conservative management of lacerations of the hand: randomized controlled trial. BMJ 2002;325:299–300.

64. Via RM. Suturing unnecessary for hand lacerations under 2 cm. J Fam Pract 2003;52(1):23–4.

65. Hattori Y, Doi K, Ikeda K, et al. A retrospective study of functional outcomes after successful replantation versus amputation closure for single fingertip amputations. J Hand Surg [Am] 2006;31:811–8.

66. Strauss EJ, Weil WM, Jordan C, et al. A prospective, randomized, controlled trial of 2-ocylcyanoacrylate versus suture repair for nail bed injuries. J Hand Surg Am 2008;33(2):250–3.

67. Richards A, Crick A, Cole R. A novel method of securing the nail following nail bed repair. Plast Reconstr Surg 1999;103(7):1983–5.
68. Hassan MS, Kannan RY, Rehman N, et al. Difficult adherent nail bed dressings: an escape route. Emerg Med J 2005;22:312.
69. Pasapula C, Strick M. The use of chloramphenicol ointment as an adhesive for replacement of the nail plate after simple nail bed repairs. J Hand Surg [Br] 2004; 29(6):634–5.
70. Roser SE, Gellman H. Comparison of nail bed repair versus nail trephination for subungual hematomas in children. J Hand Surg [Am] 1999;24:1166–70.
71. Dire DJ. Cat bite wounds: risk factors for infection. Ann Emerg Med 1991;20:973–9.
72. Chen E, Hornig S, Shepherd SM, et al. Primary closure of mammalian bites. Acad Emerg Med 2000;7:157–61.
73. Burke JF. The effective period of preventive antibiotic action in experimental incisions and dermal lesions. Surgery 1961;50:161–8.
74. Edlich RF, Kenney JG, Morgan RF, et al. Antimicrobial treatment of minor soft tissue lacerations: a critical review. Emerg Med Clin North Am 1986;4(3):561–80.
75. Sacks T. Prophylactic antibiotics in traumatic wounds. J Hosp Infect 1988;11(Suppl A):251–8.
76. Roberts AHN, Teddy PJ. A prospective trial of prophylactic antibiotics in hand lacerations. Br J Surg 1977;64:394–6.
77. Cummings P, Del Beccaro MA. Antibiotics to prevent infection of simple wounds: a meta-analysis of randomized studies. Am J Emerg Med 1995;13:396–400.
78. Whittaker JP, Nancarrow JD, Sterne GD. The role of antibiotic prophylaxis in clean incised hand injuries: a prospective randomized placebo controlled double blind trial. J Hand Surg [Br] 2005;30(2):162–7.
79. Zubowicz VN, Gravier M. Management of early human bites of the hand: a prospective randomized study. Plast Reconstr Surg 1991;88(1):111–4.
80. Stevenson J, McNaughton G, Riley J. The use of prophylactic flucloxacillin in treatment of open fractures of the distal phalanx within an accident and emergency department: a double-blind randomized placebo-controlled trial. J Hand Surg [Br] 2003;28(5):388–94.
81. Callaham M. Prophylactic antibiotics in common dog bite wounds: a controlled study. Ann Emerg Med 1980;9:410–4.
82. Wu T. Simple techniques for closing skin defects and improving cosmetic results. Aust Fam Physician 2006;35(7):492–6.
83. Lowe T, Paoloni R. Sutured wounds: factors associated with patient-rated cosmetic scores. Emerg Med Australas 2006;18(3):259–67.
84. Bar-Meir E, Zaslansky R, Regev E, et al. Nitrous oxide administered by the plastic surgeon for repair of facial lacerations in children in the emergency room. Plast Reconstr Surg 2006;117:1571–5.
85. Gassner HG, Brissett AE, Otley CC, et al. Botulinum toxin to improve facial wound healing: a prospective, blinded, placebo-controlled study. Mayo Clin Proc 2006;81(8): 1023–8.
86. Kragh JF, Basamania CJ. Surgical repair of acute traumatic closed transection of the biceps brachii. J Bone Joint Surg 2002;84-A(6):992–8.
87. Crow BD, Haltom JD, Carson WL, et al. Evaluation of a novel biomaterial for intrasubstance muscle laceration repair. J Orthop Res 2007;25:396–403.
88. Baurmash HD, Monto M. Delayed healing human bite wounds of the orofacial area managed with immediate primary closure: treatment rationale. J Oral Maxillofac Surg 2005;63:1391–7.

Wound Debridement:
Therapeutic Options and Care Considerations

Janice M. Beitz, PhD, RN, CS, CNOR, CWOCN

KEYWORDS

- Methods • Debridement methods • Healing barriers • Healing facilitators

KEY POINTS

- Wound debridement is a critical component of promoting optimal healing for a wound with necrotic tissue.
- Although much is known about the multiple barriers to healing that necrotic detritus presents, much is still unknown about the best ways, timing, and approaches to constructing a healthy wound bed.
- Future research needs to address the continuing questions and issues associated with promotion of quality chronic wound healing outcomes.

Although the topic of wound healing physiology and its critical components have been described for many years, a greater emphasis on preparation of the wound bed for optimal healing and health has pervaded the contemporary literature.[1–3] This scrutiny makes supreme sense in the context of acute and especially chronic wound healing. Necrotic tissue and other similar substances serve to impede or totally halt wound healing. A wound bed in need of debridement will not improve until this impediment is removed.

The importance of debridement has been known for centuries. Early descriptions of debridement date back to Hippocrates who described the deleterious effects of leaving necrotic tissue in wounds.[4] This article addresses the topic of wound debridement, including issues in the use of debridement, available methods, and nursing considerations associated with implementation. When available, evidence-based practice approaches and best practices will underpin the discussion.

BENEFITS OF WOUND DEBRIDEMENT

What is wound bed preparation and why is it integrally related to wound debridement? Falanga[1] defines wound bed preparation as the "global management of the wound to accelerate endogenous healing or to facilitate the effectiveness of other

A version of this article was previously published in *Nursing Clinics* 40:2.

School of Nursing, La Salle University, 1900 West Olney Avenue, Philadelphia, PA 19141, USA

E-mail address: beitz@lasalle.edu

Crit Care Nurs Clin N Am 24 (2012) 239–253

doi:10.1016/j.ccell.2012.03.009

0899-5885/12/$ – see front matter © 2012 Elsevier Inc. All rights reserved.

therapeutic measures." Wound debridement is only one component of this facilitative process. Wound bed preparation is really composed of four considerations that have been organized into the mnemonic device "TIME": *T*issue that is nonviable or deficient must be debrided. *I*nfection (or inflammation) must be reduced and managed. *M*oisture imbalance or exudate control must be addressed to avoid desiccation or maceration. *E*pidermal margins (or edges) of the wound must be examined for nonadvancement. Nonmigration of epidermal cells may signify the need for other adjunctive therapies.[5–7]

What purposes do wound debridement serve? The word itself provides a clue because debridement derives from the French (*débrider*) meaning "to unbridle" or remove a restraint.[8] The process of debridement is important for several crucial reasons: to enhance wound assessment, to decrease the potential for infection, to activate important cellular activity, and to remove physical barriers to healing (necrotic tissue).

The critical nature of quality wound assessment pervades the modern literature on wound care. Necrotic tissue prevents recognition of true wound depth, the presence of tunneling and undermining, and deep infected material. Provided adequate blood supply is present, necrotic tissue must be removed from any wound for optimal assessment.

Debridement helps to remove bacteria. Evidence suggests that significant numbers of bacteria in a wound will slow healing. When bacteria exceed 100,000 (10^5) bacteria/g of tissue, wound healing processes do not proceed normally.[9] It is unclear whether bacterial burden is a cause or consequence of impaired healing;[10] however, it is clear that necrotic matter in a wound encourages growth of anaerobic bacteria that are deleterious.

Debridement also helps to remove biofilms, which are theorized to slow wound healing. Biofilms are certain bacteria and other organisms that are covered with an extrapolysaccharide matrix. Biofilms are resistant to antibiotics and the normal immune systems of the host.[11,12]

Debriding processes may also ameliorate senescent cells. These aged cells have significantly less protein production and proliferation abilities. Debridement acts to reduce the presence of these senescent cells so that younger, healthier cells are available for wound healing. In addition, necrotic tissue leads to the release of endotoxins that inhibit keratinocytes and fibroblast activity.[12]

Another role of debridement is to remove the excess tissue that surrounds chronic wounds. Neuropathic ulcers are often associated with callus formation. Excision of the callus allows tissue-healing cells to proliferate, migrate, and ultimately heal.[2,10] Another benefit of debridement is its effect on growth factor activity. It is hypothesized that chronic wounds are lacking in these proteins or that they may be unavailable for wound healing processes because of binding to proteins present in the chronic wound.[13,14] Debridement releases activated platelets that promulgate various growth factors and cytokines.[15]

Necrotic tissue may also act to "splint" a wound; the presence of necrotic tissue can prevent closure by inhibiting wound contraction processes.[16] Conversely, if a wound closes prematurely over necrotic material, it can lead to dead space and potential abscess formation.[17]

The multiple beneficial components of debridement are critically important to optimal outcomes. If initial wound assessment is incorrect, for example, subsequent treatment will likely be problematic. A necrotic wound that is diagnosed as a pressure ulcer but is really pyoderma gangrenosum will not respond to pressure reduction but will respond to medication therapy (eg, steroids and debridement to follow as necessary). For some persons with pyoderma gangrenosum, debridement may actually worsen the inflammatory process.[18]

THE PROCESS OF WOUND HEALING: BARRIERS AND FACILITATORS

An appreciation of the importance of wound debridement is enhanced when the discussion in placed in the context of wound healing. It is especially compelling in light of wound healing in chronic wounds.

Normal wound healing (the kind associated with acute wounds) is ordinarily structured in phases. Although the phases are often discussed separately, in reality they overlap. The four phases include hemostasis, inflammation, proliferation, and remodeling. Hemostasis follows injury immediately, and the primary purpose is clot formation. A major cell present in this phase is the platelet. Inflammation targets removal of bacteria and debris and, secondarily, stimulation of cells critical for subsequent phases. The major cell of this phase is the macrophage. Proliferation is the phase in which new blood vessels grow so that granulation tissue will form. The major cells are fibroblasts and endothelial cells. In the final phase, collagen deposited in the scar strengthens tissue to improve tensile strength.

Chronic wounds do not heal in this orderly and efficient way. Rather, systemic and local factors impede normal phase progression. These chronic wounds have been called "stuck" or "stunned" wounds.[19,20] Barriers include systemic issues such as older (or very young) age, stress, malnutrition, poor tissue oxygenation, immune suppression, concomitant diseases like diabetes or cancer, medication therapy (steroids or chemotherapy), or irradiation. Local factors are also critically important, including poor perfusion, tissue edema, high bacterial burden, lack of wound moisture, use of cytotoxic agents, mechanical stressors, inappropriate wound care, and, pertinent to the current discussion, the presence of necrotic tissue. The last factor is of major importance.[21] It is not accidental that the first factor in the TIME mnemonic is tissue debridement. Nonviable or deficient tissue will impede further improvement because it will be impossible to halt infection, to keep the wound bed moisture balanced, and to help epidermal edges come together. Stated simply, gangrenous, necrotic, devitalized, and ischemic tissue need to be debrided.

Debridement is a salient component of facilitators to wound healing. These facilitators include good nutrition, wound protection, a moist wound environment, adequate oxygen supply, appropriate bioburden, and amelioration of the cause of the wound if possible. However, even in the presence of multiple facilitators, overcoming necrotic tissue in a wound bed is difficult.[22]

SPECIAL ROLE OF WOUND BED DEBRIDEMENT

The positive clinical outcome of wound debridement is a viable wound base. This viability allows for the correct functioning of growth factors and decreased inflammatory cytokines, proteases, and deleterious substances. Debridement should be distinguished from wound cleansing. Wound cleansing is used to remove foreign materials, reduce bioburden, and ameliorate odor and exudates. Topical cleansing products include antiseptics, antibiotics, detergents, surfactants, saline, and water. Wound cleansing will not effectively debride a wound that has substantial necrotic tissue.[23]

Chronic nonhealing wounds can endanger patients' well being. Bone infection (osteomyelitis), septicemia, and generalized sepsis seriously threaten patients' lives. Even without progressing to this level of severity, large chronically nonhealing wounds can lose large amounts of protein.[24]

Optimal wound debridement is based on comprehensive patient and wound assessment. For example, a necrotic pressure ulcer will not improve despite quality debridement processes if the true causative factor (pressure) is not reduced or eliminated. Experienced clinicians can attest to the fact that previously treated pressure ulcers may develop new necrotic tissue if further pressure damage ensues. Similarly, no degree of debridement will control the venous hypertension associated with venous stasis ulcers. Once basic causes are addressed effectively, debridement of the wound bed can progress. Mounting evidence supports good wound cleansing, and debridement enhances wound healing. If gentle nontoxic cleansing does not remove superficial necrotic, nonviable tissue then other debridement methods should be enacted.[25]

One caveat is noteworthy. Successful wound debridement will make a wound look bigger (and possibly worse) to nonprofessionals. The enlargement of the wound is actually promoting healing. Documentation by the wound care professional should alert clinicians and appropriate significant others that debridement will likely make a wound look as if it is deteriorating before it will eventually improve.

What does nonviable tissue look like? Necrotic tissue generally takes two forms: slough and eschar. Slough is dead tissue that is moist and stringy and yellow, tan, gray, or greenish-gray in color. Eschar is desiccated dead tissue that looks leathery and may vary from thick to thin. Eschar is most often black but can also be red or tannish brown. Both slough and eschar are attached to the wound bed.[4,26,27]

A critically important concept grounds the optimal use of debridement. Some wounds should not be debrided. An extremity ulcer with stable eschar is an example. For a limb without good blood supply, the eschar acts as a physiologic barrier to infection. The eschar should not be removed but rather protected. Likewise, a person who is at an end of life stage and has poor peripheral perfusion should likely not be subjected to invasive surgery. Not all patients with necrotic wounds need surgery before they die. Conversely, it is also central to optimal care to recognize when debridement is needed urgently. A person who has diabetes mellitus and presents with a necrotic foot ulcer that has clinical signs of infection (induration, fever, erythema, and exudate) needs surgical debridement in the immediate future.[28]

EVIDENCE-BASED PRACTICE AND WOUND DEBRIDEMENT

Traditionally, wound care and wound debridement specifically have been grounded in best practices approaches. Best practice approaches have been based on expert opinion, tradition, and anecdotal experience. In contemporary health care, best practice approaches are acceptable in areas where there is insufficient evidence to generate evidence-based guidelines.[29]

More recently, wound debridement approaches have been scrutinized, and a more rigorous evidence base is emerging. The need to remove necrotic tissue is widely accepted. Indeed, the National Guideline Clearinghouse,[30] in its recommendations for pressure ulcer treatment, stated that necrotic tissues should be debrided based on patient condition, treatment goals, and the amount of necrotic tissue in the wound bed. They gave this statement a "D4" rating, that is, the recommendation is based on existing high quality evidence-based guidelines. However, no randomized controlled trials have been conducted that examine the effect of healing of debridement versus no debridement of chronic wounds.[4] Indeed, to generate such a trial would create substantial ethical dilemmas for its researchers.

Evidence for the effectiveness of different methods of debridement is generally lacking, and methods of measurement are poorly controlled.[8] Fortunately, some controlled trials are beginning to elucidate the "best" methods in selected situations and in comparison with other methods. For example, Sherman[31] studied a cohort of 103 patients with 145 ulcers. Sixty-one of 70 patients received maggot or conventional treatment of wounds (moisture retentive dressings). He found that maggot debridement therapy was statistically significantly better in achieving greater and faster debridement than conventional therapy.

A recent Cochrane Library Review[32] examined five randomized controlled trials of debridement of diabetic foot ulcers. Three trials used hydrogel compared with two trials that used sharp debridement and one trial that used larval therapy. The pooled analysis showed that the hydrogels were significantly more effective than gauze or standard care in healing diabetic foot ulcers. Reviews such as this are extremely limited, to date. Another recent study[33] examined the efficacy of two enzymatic agents (collagenase and papain-urea) on pressure ulcer debridement. The researchers concluded that debridement was more rapid with the papain-urea formulation. In 1999, Bradley and colleagues[34] reviewed 35 randomized controlled trials and summarized the evidence for relative effectiveness of different debridement methods. The studies used dextranomer beads, cadexomer iodine, hydrogels, enzymatic agents, zinc oxide tape, surgery, or sharp debridement, and maggots. The authors concluded that evidence was insufficient to promote one debridement method over another. Steed and colleagues[35] found in a retrospective review of data on diabetics with plantar ulcers with good blood supply that frequent sharp debridement coupled with recombinant growth factor therapy had a higher rate of healing versus those patients who underwent growth factor therapy alone.

Despite recent endeavors, generally, knowledge about the optimal frequency, extent, and type of debridement is limited.[19] Systematic literature reviews of controlled clinical trials will become increasingly available from multiple sources such as the Cochrane Library and the American College of Physicians Journal Club. For the greatest level of support, systematic reviews should include only true experimental studies.[29]

One way in which these systematic reviews are linked to patient care is clinical practice guidelines. These guidelines include available research evidence such as reviews of controlled clinical trials plus other available evidence pertaining to treatment and evaluation of outcomes. These guidelines are generally broader in scope. Clinical practice guidelines for wound care are available from many sources such as the Wound, Ostomy, Continence Nurses Society (www.wocn.org), the National Guideline Clearinghouse (www.guideline.gov), and the Agency for Healthcare Research and Quality (www.ahrq.gov/clinic/epcix.htm), to name only a few.[36] Wound debridement approaches will likely become more streamlined as available systematic reviews and clinical practice guidelines guide information-seeking clinicians.

No systematic review can replace critical clinical expertise. Once clinicians determine that wound bed debridement is necessary and safe, they need to select an appropriate method or methods, cognizant of how debridement processes work and the advantages and disadvantages associated with them. In this way, correct methods can be listed to appropriate patients. A recent consensus project[5] enacted by national wound care specialists developed an algorithm to assist clinicians to choose the method of debridement matching either primary, secondary, or maintenance debridement needs.

METHODS OF WOUND DEBRIDEMENT

Multiple methods are available for wound debridement, including surgical or sharp, mechanical, chemical, autolytic, enzymatic, biotherapeutic, laser, and "other" methods.

Box 1
Factors influencing choice of wound debridement method

Amount of debris

Available time for debridement

Cost of debridement process

Nature of care setting

Patient allergies

Patient's pain level

Patient's prognosis and treatment plan

Patient's wishes and opinions

Potential patient problems

Maceration of wound

Tissue trauma

Bleeding (hemorrhage)

Presence of infection

Size of wound

Skill of the clinician

Type of debris

Type of exudate

Wound depth and undermining and tunneling

Some methods are considered "selective" in that they remove only the necrotic or devitalized tissue. Nonselective methods remove normal as well as necrotic tissue. For obvious reasons, selective methods are usually preferred. Generally, there is no one best approach. Each method is appropriate for certain clinical situations and may be used in combination effectively—and so goes the search for the ultimate debridement tool or method. Rather, the choice of debridement method depends on multiple contextual factors associated with the patient and the wound (**Box 1**). To assist with debridement method choice, various algorithms are becoming available that focus on chronic wound care.[7] However, optimal use of wound bed debridement techniques ultimately depends on education and experience. **Table 1** contains the various methods of debridement with advantages and disadvantages associated with each. An interesting phenomenon is occurring related to wound debridement methods. Older more "alternative" methods are reemerging as legitimate methods of topical therapy and debridement. These methods include biotherapy (eg, maggots) and the use of natural substances that can be categorized as "other" types of debridement, including the topical use of honey. In three recent controlled clinical trials,[37] honey was associated with faster healing in superficial burns than transparent dressings or silver sulfadiazine. Honey is also associated with autolytic debridement, deodorizing action, and an antibacterial action.

Patient and family wishes must be considered along with best available evidence. Sometimes a best practices approach is not taken because a patient does not wish aggressive (or conversely, conservative) therapy.

Table 1
Types and methods of debridement

Method/Definition	Advantages	Disadvantages	Contraindications
Surgical/Conservative Sharp Selective Use of instruments to remove necrotic tissue from wound bed. The instruments can include scalpel, forceps, and scissors	Fast and effective Selective to only necrotic tissue May be performed by specially educated nurses, therapists, and physicians Can be performed at bedside for smaller wounds Preferred method when debridement is urgently indicated (eg, sepsis)	Analgesia/anesthesia required especially for bedside usage Substantial costs included Painful Requires discernment of viable vs nonviable tissue Potential for bacteremia and sequelae Need to assess for blood dyscrasias and anticoagulant effects Requires special training and/or licensure Extensive surgical debridement requires patient's written consent Large size wounds usually require an operating room visit	Bleeding disorders Patient instability or severe immune compromise Ischemic extremity Lack of expertise in procedure Densely adherent tissue in which interface between viable and necrotic tissue is not clear With great caution in anti-coagulated patient[7,8,40–42]
Mechanical Nonselective Wet-to-dry dressings Moist saline sponge placed in wound is allowed to dry; removal of dry gauze removes devitalized tissue	Good for larger wounds with substantial devitalized assue Good for nonsurgical candidates	Painful Not cost effective; requires several daily dressing changes Non selective; removes both healthy and necrotic tissue Gauze fibers can embed in wound creating foreign body reaction Potential for maceration of surrounding skin Trauma to capillaries may cause bleeding May disperse bacteria on removal Does not provide thermal protection or bacterial barrier Dated method given other modern therapies available	Clean granulating wound[4,7,24,26,38,41,42,49,51]

(continued on next page)

Table 1
(continued)

	Advantages	Disadvantages	Indications
Hydrotherapy Also called whirlpool; Places patient in bath in which warmed swirling water softens and removes devitalized tissue	Excellent for cleansing wound and surrounding tissue Usually provides a degree of increased comfort for patient Increases circulation to wound surface	Requires patient transport May overtraumatize wound bed May macerate peri-wound skin May increase risk for waterborne infections such as *Pseudomonas aeruginosa* Requires disinfection of whirlpool tank Requires care worker protection from aerosolization via personal protective equipment Can increase venous congestion in lower extremities exacerbating venous hypertension	Clean granulating wounds Diabetics with severe neuropathy[24,26,47]
Pulsed lavage Use of specialized equipment that allows pulsating irrigation with fluid (often saline) with combined suction	Permits variation of pulsed fluid pressures (ideally 4–15 psi) Excellent for bed-bound patients	May be painful; may require premedication May drive harmful organisms deeper into tissue	Clean granulating wound[24,40]
Chemical Nonselective Hypochlorites (eg, Dakin's solution)	Helps debride necrotic slowly Lowers microbial count	Deleterious to healing tissue and wound healing cells Possible irritant effects on surrounding peri-wound skin	Clean, noninfected wounds[4,42,54]
Hydrogen peroxide	Desloughing agent Has some bactericidal effect	Deleterious to healing tissue and wound healing cells Possible irritant effects on surrounding peri-wound skin Theoretical risk of air embolism	Clean granulating wound[4]
Povidone iodine	Cheap and readily available Broad spectrum of antimicrobial activity May help dry slough for easier sharp debridement	Deleterious to fibroblasts in therapeutic dilutions Stains tissue	Clean, noninfected wound Iodine allergy[4,7,46]

Cadexomer iodine (eg, Iodosorb, Iodoflex)	Slow-release Safe for cellular viability and absorbs exudates Can absorb up to 7 times its weight Comes as ointment or dressing Helps with autolytic debridement Stimulates wound healing process	Safe for fibroblasts and other wound healing cells Used with caution in patients with thyroid disease	Clean, noninfected wound[4,26,46]
Autolytic Selective Use of body's own wound fluid enzymes to liquefy necrotic tissue; accomplished through moisture-retentive topical therapy. Some types fully occlude whereas others are semi-occlusive Hydrocolloids, act to retain body's own moisture in wound	Safe and slowly effective Patient comfort, usually soothing by covering open nerve endings Associated with decreased risk of wound infection Indicated when no urgent clinical need for drainage or removal of revitalized tissue Good choice for patients who are not surgical candidates Easy to perform Performed in any care setting	Works slowly compared with other methods Cannot be used in certain situations (eg, occlusive dressing over eschar in pulseless extremity or infected wound) Requires constant monitoring of wound for infection in immune-compromised patients Must assess blood supply in extremity Hydrocolloid dressing fluid odor often mistaken for "infected"	Infected ulcers or wounds Cellulitic wounds Severe neutropenia Deep extensive wound With great caution in immune compromised and frail elderly[4,7,24,26,30,41,42,52]
Hydrogels, donate water into necrotic tissue to liquefy it Alginates Foam Hydrofiber Moisture vapor permeable, transparent, film, retains body's own moisture in wound	Hydrogels, alginates, foams and hydrofibers will absorb some wound fluid Maintain moist wound therapy All except for moisture vapor permeable dressings can be used in deep extensive wounds to good effect	Absorptive dressings can dry out wound bed if not discontinued when appropriate	Dry wound bed not appropriate for absorptive dressings[4,7,24,26,30,41,42,52]

(continued on next page)

Table 1
(continued)

	Selective (Advantages)	Disadvantages	Allergies/Precautions
Enzymatic Selective Protein agents (enzymes) that work by degrading and debriding necrotic tissue by digesting and dissolving it Types available include: Collagenase (Santyl) Papain-urea (Accuzyme) Papain-urea and chlorophyllin (Panafil)	Safe for patient use if used according to directions Good for settings with no sharp debridement available Good for patients receiving anticoagulants Good for patients who have contraindications to surgery Decrease wound trauma Good for home care patient Cost effective if used properly Selectively removes necrotic tissue Will not harm normal tissue Sometimes used with topical antibiotics (not always evidence-based) Can be used in infected wounds	Usually not effective for advanced cellulitic wounds Require physician or prescriber's order Slower and less aggressive than sharp debridement Cannot be used with other common wound products such as metal ions (eg, Silvadene) or with topical antiseptics (eg, Dakin's solution) Some agents require or recommend cross-hatching of eschar with a scalpel Expensive Sometimes associated with peri-wound inflammation Temporary burning sensation Knowing when to stop therapy Papain-urea has been associated rarely with anaphylaxis	Clean granulating wound Allergies Use papain-urea type agent with great caution in latex allergy patient[1,4,7,19,24,41,43,45,48]
Biotherapy Selective Also called maggot debridement therapy or biosurgery Use of sterile maggots for debriding wounds Uses larvae of *Lucilia sericata* (greenbottle fly); maggots secrete proteolytic enzymes that break down tissue	Removes only necrotic tissue Relatively inexpensive Painless Acts relatively rapidly Can be used on all ages of patients Can be used on immobilized persons and pregnant women Can be used concurrently with antibiotics Has multiple indications including: pressure ulcers, vascular ulcers, diabetic ulcers, traumatic and post surgical wounds, burns, and methicillin-resistant *S. aureus*-infected wounds	Some patients find too offensive to accept, "yuck factor" Potential for allergic reaction Cannot use in tunneling wounds Ineffective for osteomyelitis Secretions irritate healthy skin Increased pain with use in ischemic wounds Dressing change is time consuming	Patient with allergies to eggs, soybeans, and fly larvae Lack of wound hemostasis Adhesive allergies Deep tracked wounds[41,43–46,55,56]

Method	Benefits	Disadvantages	Contraindications
Wound VAC (hypobaric therapy) Selective A sub-atmospheric pressure dressing that creates a closed wound system-applies 125 mm Hg of pressure	Removes interstitial fluid/edema Assists with granulation Acts to liquefy and remove slough and soften eschar Decreases bacterial count Can grow granulation tissue over bone and tendon	Can be painful Expensive Can cause pressure necrosis if not applied skillfully Requires electrical supply	Hemorrhage Exposed blood vessels High output enteric fistula[40,47]
Laser Selective	Debrides only necrotic tissue Decreases edema by sealing lymphatics May stimulate wound healing	Requires special equipment Requires patient and user protective gear	Clean granulating wound[17,25]
Other Selective Topical Substances Honey Use of medicinal honey usually applied by special dressings	Debrides necrotic tissues through osmotic effect of sugar Has broad spectrum antibacterial like effect Has deodorizing anti-inflammatory and anti-scarring effects Used on variety of wound including: burns, surgical wounds, necrotizing fasciitis, and chronic ulcers Cheap Not painful Can be used across care settings	May require operating room visit Slower debridement Rare adverse allergic reactions Transient stinging sensation	None reported[37,50,53]

Data from Refs. 1,4,7,8,17,19,24,26,30,37,38,40–56

Quality patient education and cultural competence and sensitivity play critical roles in the use of debridement approaches. In today's multicultural society, caregivers must be cognizant of ethnic and religious preferences. In the author's experience, patients or caregivers may be uncooperative with debridement approaches based on erroneous interpretations or perceptions. For example, a patient and his family initially refused an enzymatic debriding process because they thought it contained substances proscribed by their religion. Another patient feared a negative pressure wound device because it would injure (electrically shock) him. Both patients agreed to therapy when full processes and ingredients were explained and documentation was shared.

Another component of patient education regarding debridement is the need for ongoing debridement in chronic wounds.[20] Maintenance debridement is necessary in chronic wounds in which the underlying pathology is associated with continuous recurrence of slough and eschar. Patients need to be counseled that continuing debridement does not constitute treatment failure or poor patient compliance.

Although the armamentarium of wound debridement methods has expended substantially, recent research[38] has substantiated that the most traditional, cost ineffective method, saline wet to dry gauze, persists in being the most commonly used approach even in circumstances for which there is little evidence to support its use (clean open surgical wounds healing by secondary intention). These researchers and other authors suggest that tradition, lack of education, and poor understanding of cost efficacy drive many physicians' debridement choices.[39]

SUMMARY

Wound debridement is a critical component of promoting optimal healing for a wound with necrotic tissue. Although much is known about the multiple barriers to healing that necrotic detritus presents, much is still unknown about the best ways, timing, and approaches to constructing a healthy wound bed. Falanga's[2] "black box," a metaphor for the unknown components of wound healing and debridement, should remind all practitioners that future research needs to address the continuing questions and issues associated with promotion of quality chronic wound healing outcomes.

SUGGESTED READING

Armstrong DG, Lavery LA, Masquez JR, et al. How and why to surgically debride neuropathic diabetic foot wounds. JAPMA 2002;92(7):402–4.

Ashworth J. Conservative sharp debridement: the professional and legal issues. Prof Nurse 2002;17(10):585–8.

Brown GS. Reporting outcomes for stage IV pressure ulcer healing: a proposal. Adv Skin Wound Care 2000;13:277–83.

Campton-Johnston S, Wilson J. Infected wound management: advanced technologies, moisture-retentive dressings, and die-hard methods. Crit Care Nurs Q 2001; 24(2):64–77.

Capasso VA, Munro BH. The cost and efficacy of two wound treatments. AORN J 2003;77(5):984–1004.

Copson D. Evaluating a new technique for the treatment of chronic wounds. Prof Nurse 2000;17(12):729–33.

Dharmarajan TS, Ahmed S. The growing problems of pressure ulcers. Postgrad Med 2003;113(5):77–85.

Falabella A. Debridement of wounds. Wounds 1998;10:1C–9.

Fink A, Deluca G. Necrotizing fasciitis: pathophysiology and treatment. Medsurg Nurs 2003;11(1):33–6.

Hahn JF, Olsen CL, Tomaselli N, et al. Wounds: nursing care and product selection: part II. Nursing Spectrum Career Fitness Online 2002. Available at: http://www.nursing spectrum.com/ce/ce81.html. Accessed December 27, 2003.

Harding K, Cutting K, Price P. The cost effectiveness of wound management protocols of care. Br J Nurs 2000;9(19):S4–24.

Hawkins-Bradley B, Walden M. Treatment of a non-healing wound with hypergranulation tissue and rolled edges. J Wound Ostomy Continence Nurs 2002;29(6):320–4.

Holloway S, Ryder J. Management of a patient with postoperative necrotizing fasciitis. Br J Nurs 2002;11(16):525–32.

Morison MJ. A framework for patient assessment and care planning. In: Morison MJ, Ovington L, Wilkie K, editors. Chronic wound care: a problem based learning approach. Edinburgh: CV Mosby; 2004. p. 46–66.

Wound Ostomy Continence Nurses Society. Position statement: conservative sharp wound debridement for registered nurses 1996. Available at: http://www.wocn.org/publications/posstate/debride.html. Accessed December 27, 2003.

REFERENCES

1. Falanga V. Wound bed preparation and the role of enzymes: a case for multiple action of therapeutic agents. Wounds 2002;14(2):47–57.

2. Falanga V. Wound bed preparation: future approaches. Ostomy Wound Manage 2003;49(5ASuppl):S30–3.

3. Kirsner R. Wound bed preparation. Ostomy Wound Manage 2003;49(5A)(Suppl): S2–3.

4. O'Brien M. Exploring methods of wound debridement. Br J Community Nurs 2003; 7(Suppl 1):S10–8.

5. Ayello E, Dowsett C, Schultz G, et al. Time heals all wounds. Nursing 2004;34(4): 36–42.

6. Sibbald RG, Orsted H, Schultz GS, et al. For the international wound bed preparation advisory board and the Canadian chronic wound advisory board. Preparing the wound bed 2003: focus on infection and inflammation. Ostomy Wound Manage 2003;49(11):24–51.

7. Sibbald RG, Williamson D, Orsted HL, et al. Preparing the wound bed–debridement, bacterial balance, and moisture balance. Ostomy Wound Manage 2000; 46(11):14–35.

8. Leaper D. Sharp technique for wound debridement. World Wide Wounds. Available at: http://www.worldwidewounds.com/2002/december/leaper/sharp-debridement. html. Accessed February 6, 2004.

9. Robson MC, Stenberg BD, Heggers JP. Wound healing alterations caused by infection. Clin Plast Surg 1990;17:485–92.

10. Zacur H, Kirsner RS. Debridement: rationale and therapeutic options. Wounds 2002;14(Suppl 7):S25–65.

11. Serralta VW, Harrison-Balestra C, Cazzaniga AL, et al. Lifestyles of bacteria in wounds: presence of biofilms? Wounds 2001;13(1):29–34.

12. Wysocki AB. Evaluating and managing open skin wounds: colonization versus infection. AACN Clin Issues 2002;13(3):382–97.

13. Kerstein MD, Reis ED. Current surgical perspectives in wound healing. Wounds 2001;13(2):53–8.

14. Mulder GD, Vandeberg JS. Cellular senescence and matrix metalloprotease activity in chronic wounds. JAPMA 2002;92(1):34–7.

15. Hunt TK, Hopf H, Hussain Z. Physiology of wound healing. Adv Skin Wound Care 2000;13(Suppl 2):S6–11.

16. Baharestani M. The clinical relevance of debridement. In: Baharestani M, Gottrup F, Holstein P, et al, editors. The clinical relevance of debridement. Berlin: Springer-Verlag; 1999. p. 1–6.

17. Dolynchuk K. Debridement. In: Krasner DL, Rodeheaver GT, Sibbald RG, editors. Chronic wound care: a clinical sourcebook for healthcare professionals. 3rd edition. Wayne (PA): HMP Communication; 2001. p. 385–90.

18. Chakrabarty A, Phillips T. Diagnostic dilemmas in pyoderma gangrenosum. Wounds 2002;14:302–5.

19. Ennis WJ, Meneses P. Wound healing at the local level: the stunned wound. Ostomy Wound Manage 2000;46(IA):395–485.

20. Schultz G, Sibbald RG, Falanga V, et al. Wound bed preparation: a systematic approach to wound management. Wound Repair Regen 2003;11:1–20.

21. Hall P, Schumann L. Wound care: meeting the challenge. J Am Acad Nurse Pract 2001;13(6):258–68.

22. Stotts N, Wipke-Tevis D. Co-factors in impaired wound healing. In: Krasner DL, Rodeheaver GT, Sibbald RG, editors. Chronic wound care: a clinical sourcebook for healthcare professionals. Wayne (PA): HMP Communications; 2001. p. 265–72.

23. Ovington LG, Eisenbud D. Dressings and cleansing agents. In: Morison MJ, Ovington L, Wilkie K, editors. Chronic wound care: a problem-based learning approach. Edinburgh: CV Mosby; 2004. p. 117–28.

24. Ayello E, Cuddigan J, Kerstein M. Skip the knife: debriding wounds without surgery. Nursing 2002;32(9):58–63.

25. Dolynchuk K, Keast D, Campbell K, et al. Best practices for the prevention and treatment of pressure ulcers. Ostomy Wound Manage 2000;46(11):38–52.

26. Nelson D, Dilloway MA. Principles, products, and practical aspects of wound care. Crit Care Nurs Q 2002;25(1):33–54.

27. Tong A. Recognizing, managing and removing slough. NT Plus 2000;96(29):15–6.

28. Krasner DL. How to prepare the wound bed. Ostomy Wound Manage 2001;47(4): 59–61.

29. Gray M, Beitz J, Colwell J, et al. Evidence-based nursing practice II: advanced concepts for WOC nursing practice. J Wound Ostomy Continence Nurs 2004;31(2): 53–61.

30. Singapore Ministry of Health. Nursing management of pressure ulcers in adults. Singapore: Ministry of Health. 2001. Available at: http://www.guideline.gov/summary/summary.aspx?doc_id=3276.html. Accessed January 28, 2004.

31. Sherman RA. Maggot versus conservative debridement therapy for the treatment of pressure ulcers. Wound Repair Regen 2002;10(4):208.

32. Smith J. Debridement of diabetic foot ulcers [abstract]. Cochrane Library. Chichester (UK): Wiley & Sons; 2003. p. 4.

33. Alvarez OM, Fernandez-Obregon A, Rogers RS, et al. Chemical debridement of pressure ulcers: a prospective, randomized, comparative trial of collagenase and papain/urea formulations. Wounds 2000;12(12):15–25.

34. Bradley M, Cullum N, Sheldon T. The debridement of chronic wounds: a systematic review. Health Tech Assess 1999;3(17 Pt 1):iii–iv, 1–78.

35. Steed DL, Donohue D, Webster MW. Effect of extensive debridement and treatment on the healing of diabetic foot ulcers. J Am Coll Surg 1996;183:61–4.

36. Ryan S, Perrier L, Sibbald RG. Searching for evidence-based medicine in wound care: an introduction. Ostomy Wound Manage 2003;49(11):67–75.

37. Molan P. Re-introducing honey in the management of wounds and ulcers–theory and practice. Ostomy Wound Manage 2002;48(11):28–40.

38. Armstrong M, Price P. Wet-to-dry gauze dressings: fact and fiction. Wounds 2004; 16(2):56–62.
39. Van Rijswijk L, Beitz J. The traditions and terminology of wound dressings: food for thought. J Wound Ostomy Continence Nurs 1998;25(3):116–22.
40. Attinger CE, Bulan E, Blume PA. Surgical debridement: the key to successful wound healing and reconstruction. Clin Podiatr Med Surg 2000;17(4):599–630.
41. Ayello E, Baranoski S, Kerstein M, et al. Wound debridement. In: Baranoski S, Ayello E, Wound care essentials: practice principles. Philadelphia: Lippincott, Williams & Wilkins; 2003. p. 117–26.
42. Burns P. Wound bed preparation: essentials for wound care-debridement, bacterial balance, and exudate management. The Remington Report 2003;May/June:7–9.
43. Claxton MJ, Armstrong DG, Short B, et al. 5 questions and answers about maggot debridement therapy. Adv Skin Wound Care 2003;16(2):99–102.
44. Dossey L. Maggots and leeches: when science and aesthetics collide. Altern Ther Health Med 2002;8(4):12–6, 106.
45. Drisdelle R. Maggot debridement therapy. Nursing 2003;33(6):17
46. Drosou A, Falabella A, Kirsner RS. Antiseptics on wounds: an area of controversy. Wounds 2003;15(5):149–66.
47. Hess CL, Howard MA, Attinger CE. A review of mechanical adjuncts in wound healing: hydrotherapy, ultrasound, negative pressure, therapy, hyperbaric oxygen, and electrostimulation. Ann Plast Surg 2003;51(2):210–8.
48. Hewitt H, Wint Y, Talabere L, et al. The use of papaya on pressure ulcers: a natural alternative. Am J Nurs 2002;102(12):73–7.
49. Lee SK, Turnbull GB. Wound care: What's really cost effective? Nursing Homes Long-Term Care Management 2001;50(4):40–4, 74–5.
50. Molan P. Honey as a topical antibacterial agent for treatment of infected wounds. World Wide Wounds. Available at: http://www.worldwidewounds.com/2001/november/molan/honey-as-topical-agent.html. Accessed February 6, 2004.
51. Ovington L. Hanging wet to dry dressings out to dry. Adv Skin Wound Care 2002; 15(2):79–84.
52. Ovington LG. Wound care products: how to choose. Home Healthc Nurse 2001; 19(4):224–32.
53. Pieper B, Caliri M. Nontraditional wound care: a review of the evidence for the use of sugar, papaya/papain, and fatty acids. J Wound Ostomy Continence Nurs 2003;30: 175–83.
54. Stotts N. Wound infection: diagnosis and management. In: Morison MJ, Ovington L, Wilkie K, editors. Chronic wound care: a problem-based learning approach. Edinburgh: CV Mosby; 2004. p. 101–16.
55. Thomas S. The use of sterile maggots in wound management. NT Plus 2002;98(36): 45–6.
56. Thomas S, Jones M. Wound debridement: evaluating the costs. Nurs Stand 2001; 15(22):59–61.

Wound Healing Agents

Samuel B. Adams Jr, MD[a], Vani J. Sabesan, MD[b],
Mark E. Easley, MD[b],*

KEYWORDS

- Wound healing • Diabetes • Hyperbaric oxygen • Impregnated gauze
- Hydrocolloids

KEY POINTS

- This report presents a review of the process of wound healing and influencing factors, including the common products used as adjuncts to the healing process.
- A greater understanding of the alterations in diabetes mellitus allows selection of optimal wound healing agents to provide a more optimistic approach to wound closure for this large population of diabetics.
- With newer innovations such as the use of negative pressure dressings and HBO therapy, the treatment of diabetic wounds continues to improve.

When not properly treated, wounds of the foot and ankle can be devastating for both the patient and physician. Therefore, it is important to recognize treatment options best suited for a particular wound, as well as the underlying factors involved in preventing a wound from healing.

The most common impediments to wound healing include wound hypoxia, infection, presence of debris and necrotic tissue, nutritional deficiencies, inhibitory medications, and metabolic disorders such as diabetes mellitus.[1] Only before minimization of these factors will wound healing agents be effective. Diabetes mellitus is a complex metabolic disorder that affects healing of wounds directly and indirectly. Specifically, diabetes causes alterations in microvasculature, nerve function, and the immune system.

There are a multitude of wound healing agents available, with some correlation to the type of wound or underlying disease, but for the most part the use of these agents is based on inherited common practice, personal preference, or marketing activities. Currently, the medical literature is replete of high-quality, randomized, controlled trials pertaining to wound healing agents, especially in the setting of diabetes mellitus.

A version of this article was previously published in *Foot and Ankle Clinics* 11:4.
[a] Division of Orthopaedic Surgery, Duke University Medical Center, Box 2887, Durham, NC 27710, USA; [b] Division of Orthopaedic Surgery, Duke University Medical Center, Box 2950, Durham, NC 27710, USA
* Corresponding author.
E-mail address: easle004@mc.duke.edu

Crit Care Nurs Clin N Am 24 (2012) 255–260
doi:10.1016/j.ccell.2012.03.010
0899-5885/12/$ – see front matter © 2012 Elsevier Inc. All rights reserved.

Therefore, it is the goal of this article to educate the orthopedic surgeon on the proper use of wound healing agents that can be applied to foot and ankle wounds.

STAGES OF WOUND HEALING

Wound healing occurs in three phases that are not distinct and separate but more a continuum of the entire process. The first phase or inflammatory phase begins immediately after the time of injury and lasts approximately 4 days. The initial goal of this phase is hemostasis and is performed through smooth muscle contraction and subsequent occlusion of the larger damaged blood vessels. The second goal of the inflammatory phase is the removal of bacteria, foreign debris, and other contaminants. Neutrophils migrate from surrounding microvasculature to accomplish this phase after which macrophages take over. Macrophages are the predominant cell in the second stage or proliferative stage of healing. Macrophages appear 48 hours after injury at the wound site to aggressively remove necrotic tissue and foreign debris in addition to initiating two important aspects of healing, angiogenesis and fibroplasia. The proliferative or fibroblastic phase can last weeks (approximately 3 to 21 days). The neovasculature, along with collagen and proteoglycan ground substance, form granulation tissue, which fills in wound defects and increases wound tensile strength between 5 and 15 days postinjury. This is followed by the process of re-epithelialization. A moist wound surface facilitates epithelial migration. The final phase of wound healing is the maturation or remodeling phase, which begins approximately 21 days postinjury and can continue up to 1 to 2 years. Remodeling is performed by collagenases that are secreted to help debulk and reorganize collagen bundles into a more parallel arrangement. With wound contraction, this produces an increase in wound tensile strength, which is maximal at the end of the maturation phase and 80% of the original uninjured tissue's strength.

IMPEDIMENTS TO WOUND HEALING

As previously mentioned, there are several factors that can impede wound healing. Local tissue hypoxia is detrimental to all wound healing and may be the inciting event to chronic wounds, including diabetic foot and pressure ulcers.[1] Initially, hypoxia is beneficial to wound healing because it stimulates fibroblast proliferation and angiogenesis, but chronic hypoxia inhibits fibroblast replication and collagen production as well as predisposing the wound to bacterial invasion. Tobacco abuse, diabetes mellitus, peripheral vascular disease, and poor cardiac output are some of the concomitant factors that predispose a wound to tissue hypoxia.

A major impediment to wound healing is bacterial overgrowth. It has been reported that the number of bacteria needed to cause a wound infection is 10^5 bacteria per gram of tissue for most bacteria.[2] The mechanism of impairment of wound healing accomplished by bacteria is thought to be through the release of enzymes and metalloproteinases that degrade fibrin and inhibit growth factors.[3] Therefore, if infection is thought to be inhibiting wound healing, then debridement of bacteria and nonviable tissue should be undertaken. Debridement restores the host's natural balance of defense agents to bacteria, reduces the load of bacterial byproducts, and stimulates the production of local growth factors for healing.

Chronic diseases, as well as their medical therapies, can both significantly impede wound healing. Diabetes mellitus is a terrible disease that can predispose a surgical wound to poor healing potential or be the underlying etiology for the development of a foot ulcer. It is estimated that people with diabetes have a 12% to 25% lifetime risk of foot ulcer development.[4] Interventions such as glycemic control, ensuring adequate perfusion, and infection control are crucial to the management of diabetic patients with chronic wounds.

Nutritional deficiencies are also detrimental to wound healing. Serum albumin levels less than 2 g/dL have been associated with decreased wound healing from decreased fibroplasias, neovascularization, cell synthesis, and wound remodeling.[1] Additionally, it has been reported that after only 4 weeks of inadequate nutrition, phagocyte activity and lymphocyte function are diminished.[5]

WOUND HEALING AGENTS
Impregnated Gauze

Impregnated gauze are probably the most commonly used primary layer dressing on postsurgical and newly diagnosed wounds. They were developed at least as early as World War I to create a nonadherent barrier with variable occlusivity between the wound or incision and the rest of the dressing. Their ability to be nonadherent provides for increased patient comfort with dressing removal. They are composed typically of a fine mesh impregnated with a petrolatum emulsion or similar substance, as well as additives such as povidone-iodine, silver, bismuth, scarlet red, and aloe vera.[6] Adaptic (Johnson & Johnson Medical Inc., Arlington, TX, USA) is a commonly used dressing impregnated solely with petrolatum. It has an open mesh design that allows it to be completely nonocclusive. It therefore can be used on heavily draining wounds with an absorptive overlying layer, preventing maceration. Another commonly used impregnated dressing, but occlusive in nature, is Xeroform (Sparta Surgical Corp, Hayward, CA, USA). Xeroform has a petrolatum component but, in addition, has 3% bismuth tribromophenate, which acts as a mild astringent and deodorizer.[7] It should be used on wounds with minimal drainage, and is used typically as the initial layer on postoperative incisions. Additional applications include minimally draining graft sites and burns.[7] Betadine antiseptic gauze (The Purdue Frederick Company, Norwalk, CO, USA) is, as its name implies, impregnated with povidone-iodine solution instead of petrolatum. This dressing is used for contaminated or superficially infected wounds but should not be used on postoperative wounds as the cytotoxicity to new, fragile, or granulating tissue is well documented.[7]

Other Nonadherent Dressings

It is important to briefly mention another type of nonadherent dressing that is used commonly but lacks petrolatum impregnation. These dressings are composed of two or more layers, one of which is a porous inner layer to allow exudate passage, and an outer layer that is absorbent.[7] They are best suited for weaping superficial wounds (ruptured bullae, abrasion, ulcers) to prevent maceration and allow the exudate to aid in adherence prevention, because they are not quite as nonadherent as petrolatum impregnated gauze. Examples of these dressings include Telfa (Kendall Health Care Products, Mansfield, IA, USA) and Release (Johnson & Johnson Medical Inc.).

Hydrogels

Hydrogels are three-dimensional networks of hydrophilic polymers made from gelatin, polysaccharides, polyacrylamides, and sometimes other polymers.[6] These dressings come in the form of a gelatinous sheet or an amorphous wound filler.[7] The molecular nature of hydrogels allows them to retain fluid, allowing them to either absorb wound exudates or desorb chemical agents into the wound. Arguably, their ability to desorb is much greater than their ability to absorb, so these dressings should not be used on highly exudative wounds, because maceration may occur.[7] In fact, it is their ability to desorb saline or water that allows them to be used to hydrate desiccated eschars or dry skin. Hydrogels can be used on superficial acute or chronic wounds. Two examples of hydrogels include Curasol (Healthpoint Medical, Arlington, TX, USA) and DuoDerm Gel (ConvaTec, Skillman, NJ, USA).

Hydrocolloids

Hydrocolloids are composite sheets of an adhesive inner layer, a hydrophilic polymer, and a water-resistant outer layer. They differ from hydrogels in that they are much more absorptive. The wound exudates interact with the hydrophilic polymer forming a gel that expands into the wound cavity. The increased volume of gel actually enables the hydrocolloid dressing to act as a pressure dressing. Thomas and colleagues[8] reported a 50% decrease in exudate production owing to the pressure dressing effect of hydrocolloids in venous stasis ulcers.

The composite structure of hydrocolloids allows them to be a complete and waterproof dressing. Patients may shower, and depending on the amount of exudate, the dressing can be changed every 1 to 7 days.[7] The occlusivity of these dressings makes them less than ideal for infected wounds. Hydrocolloids are best suited for mild to moderately draining wounds without signs of infection or wounds where autolytic debridement of necrotic tissue is desired.[7]

Calcium Alginate

Calcium alginates are naturally occurring mixed salts of alginic acid found in seaweed. They are fibrous in nature and come in various forms including ribbons, pads, and flat dressings,[9] allowing them to be used to pack various types of wounds. Like hydrocolloids, alginates function to absorb exudate. They form a gel as exudate is absorbed through a reaction of the sodium ions from the exudate and the calcium ions in the alginate.[9] The gel nature of alginates provides additional wound packing and a moist environment for wound healing, but these dressings do require additional overlying dressing material to keep the gelatinous mass at the wound. Alginates may be able to aid in infection control. Bowler and colleagues[10] in a simulated wound study, found that alginates effectively removed bacteria from the wound fluid by trapping them in the dense fibers and gel.

Silver

Silver in various forms has been used for medical purposes for thousands of years.[11] Traditionally, it has been used as a burn dressing, but more recently, newer silver dressings have crossed over into the general wound dressing arena. Silver has a broad range of antimicrobial activity against aerobes, anaerobes, gram-negative and positive bacteria, yeast, fungi, viruses, and even methicillin and vancomycin resistant Staphylococcus aureus . There are very few side effects from topical silver therapy; silver toxicity and argyrosis are the most severe, but these are reported to resolve with cessation of therapy.[12] Silver for dressing purposes comes in many forms, and the most common are creams and sheets. Flumazine (Smith & Nephew, Largo, FL, USA) and Silvazine (Smith & Nephew) are 1% silver sulphadiazine creams with the exception of Silvazine having the additional component of 0.2% chlorhexidine digluconate. Acticoat (Smith & Nephew) is a new nanocrystalline silver dressing available in sheet form. It is composed of the silver-coated mesh and a rayon/polyester core that helps maintain wound moisture. The nanocrystalline nature of the silver provides rapid and sustained release of silver to the wound. The Acticoat dressing must be kept moist with sterile water and can be changed every 3 to 7 days. Silver dressings are not complete dressings in themselves and usually require an additional layer to keep them localized to the wound. They are suited for a variety of wounds including burns and infected superficial ulcers. They would not be suited for heavily draining wounds, as maceration may occur.

Vacuum-Assisted Closure

Negative pressure vacuum techniques in the treatment of difficult wounds have been well described in the plastic surgery literature. The technique is designed to remove chronic edema and enhance localized blood flow to increase granulation tissue, which may expedite healing. Both retrospective and prospective studies have found improved wound healing and decreased length of time to full healing with negative pressure wound dressings. A study by Clare and Fitzgibbons[13] reviewed wound vacuum treatment in 17 diabetic patients with nonhealing wounds of the lower extremity, all of whom did not respond to previous treatments with serial wound debridements and dressing changes. Although many of these patients had previous surgical interventions including irrigation and debridements and amputations, 14 of these patients successfully healed their wounds in 8.2 weeks with wound vacuum therapy. From the patients who did not respond, investigators concluded that perhaps smaller forefoot wounds and large wounds in patients with severe peripheral vascular disease may be better treated by other modalities based on the three patients who did not respond in their study. Another study by Mendonca et al.[14] found similar results in patients with diabetic foot ulcers treated with wound vacuum therapy had satisfactory healing in 13 of 18 patients at an average of 2.5 months, and it decreased wound size from 7.41 cm^2 to 1.58 cm^2. A small, randomized, prospective review by Eginton and colleagues[15] found decrease in wound depth and volume for vacuum-treated large diabetic foot wounds compared with moist gauze dressings. Although more studies are needed to delineate appropriate patient selection for successful vacuum treatment as well and more data on results of vacuum therapy, initial reports appear to support vacuum therapy as an extremely useful healing agent for chronic foot wound or ulcers in patients with diabetes or peripheral vascular disease.

Hyperbaric Oxygen Therapy

Hyperbaric oxygen (HBO) therapy allows patients to breathe 100% oxygen in a chamber with increased barometric pressure. With enhanced oxygen delivery, increased arterial oxygen tensions provide an enhanced gradient for diffusion. Additionally HBO therapy decreases tissue edema. The high oxygen concentrations act as a direct vascular smooth muscle contractile stimulus causing arterial vasoconstriction. This may seem deleterious, but the high oxygen content of the blood compensates for any reduction in blood flow, and simultaneous increase in upstream arterial resistance in combination with decreased capillary hydrostatic pressures results in resorption of fluid and decreased tissue edema. Another beneficial effect of HBO is enhanced leukocyte function. Polymorphonuclear leukocytes generate oxidative bursts that are lethal to ingested bacteria and substrate limited by oxygen. Finally, with HBO therapy, there is a decrease in oxidate free radicals and mitigation of no-reflow process. Both in vitro and in vivo studies have found positive healing effects using HBO therapy.

SUMMARY

This report presented a review of the process of wound healing as well as influencing factors in the process such as wound healing agents. A greater understanding of the alterations in diabetes mellitus allows selection of optimal wound healing agents to provide a more optimistic approach to wound closure for this large population of diabetics. We have reviewed some of the most common products used as adjuncts to the healing process. With newer innovations such as the use of negative pressure dressings and HBO therapy, the treatment of diabetic wounds continues to improve. With the increased number of wound healing agents, it is important to consider the type of wound and the conditions present when selecting one healing agent over another.

REFERENCES

1. Stadelmann WK, Digenis AG, Tobin GR. Impediments to wound healing. Am J Surg 1998;176(Suppl 2A):39S–47S.
2. Robson MC. Infection in the surgical patient: an imbalance in the normal equilibrium. Clin Plast Surg 1979;6:493–503.
3. Robson MC, Senberg BD, Heggers JD. Wound healing alterations caused by bacteria. Clin Plast Surg 1990;3:485–92.
4. Singh N, Armstrong DG, Lipsky BA. Preventing foot ulcers in patients with diabetes. JAMA 2005;293:217–28.
5. Robson MC, Burns BF, Phillips LG. Wound repair: principles and applications. In: Ruberg RL, Smith DJ, editors. Plastic surgery: a core curriculum. St. Louis (MO): Mosby; 1994. p. 3–30.
6. Ladin DA. Understanding dressings. Clin Plast Surg 1998;25(3):433–41.
7. Hanna JR, Giacopelli JA. A review of wound healing and wound dressing products. J Foot Ankle Surg 1997;36(1):2–14.
8. Thomas S, Fear M, Humphries J, et al. The effect of dressings on the production of exudates from venous leg ulcers. Wounds 1996;8:145–50.
9. Pulman K. Dressings in the management of open surgical wounds. Br J Periop Nursing 2004;14(8):354–60.
10. Bowler PG, Jones SA, Davies BJ, et al. Infection control properties of some wound dressings. J Wound Care 1999;8(10):499–502.
11. Dowsett C. An overview of Acticoat dressing in wound management. Br J Nurs 2003;12(19):S44–9.
12. Hollinger MA. Toxicological apects of topical silver pharmaceuticals. Crit Rev Toxicol 1996;26:255–60.
13. Clare MP, Fitzgibbons TC, McMullen ST, et al. Experience with the vacuum assisted closure negative pressure technique in the treatment of non-healing diabetic and dysvascular wounds. Foot Ankle Int 2002;23(10):896–901.
14. Mendonca DA, Cosker T, Makwana NK. Vacuum-assisted closure to aid wound healing in foot and ankle surgery. Foot Ankle Int 2005;26(9):761–6.
15. Eginton MT, Brown KR, Seabrook GR, et al. A prospective randomized evaluation of negative-pressure wound dressings for diabetic foot wounds. Ann Vasc Surg 2003; 17(6):645–9.

Management of Forearm Compartment Syndrome

Jeffrey B. Friedrich, MD[a], Alexander Y. Shin, MD[b],*

KEYWORDS

- Volkmann's ischemic contracture • Fasciotomy • Surgical techniques • Forearm
- Compartment syndrome

KEY POINTS

- Forearm compartment syndrome is a potentially calamitous problem that can befall persons with either injuries or external compression of the forearm.
- The absolute necessities for a good outcome are early suspicion of forearm compartment syndrome and expeditious surgical intervention.
- One must be acutely aware of the prospect of compartment syndrome in the settings of forearm diaphysis and distal radius fractures.
- Delays in diagnosis and surgical intervention can lead to ischemic contracture of the forearm that can be manifested in varying degrees but ultimately can lead to greatly diminished function of the affected upper extremity.

Forearm compartment syndrome is an entity that has been noted with a variety of injuries, external compression, and other etiologies, and if left untreated can lead to devastating complications. The final state of these complications has been traditionally given the eponym of Volkmann's ischemic contracture, and can have varying degrees of severity.[1–3] Many authors have reported a variety of etiologies for forearm compartment syndrome ranging from the common to the unusual. Some of the more relatively frequent causes of forearm compartment syndrome include supracondylar humerus fractures in pediatric patients as well as distal radius fractures in adult and pediatric patients.[4–6] Other authors have reported more unusual etiologies including complicated Bier blocks, malfunctioning pneumatic tourniquets with elective hand surgery, spider bites, industrial vacuum accidents, ring avulsions, a variety of intravenous line extravasations, injection of illicit drugs, hematomas as a result of anticoagulation, inadvertent administration of intravenous hypertonic

A version of this article was previously published in *Hand Clinics* 23:2.
[a] Department of Surgery and Orthopedics, University of Washington, Harborview Medical Center, 8th Floor, East Hospital, Box 359835 325 Ninth Avenue, Seattle, WA 98104, USA;
[b] Division of Hand Surgery, Department of Orthopedic Surgery, Mayo Clinic, 200 First Street, SW, Rochester, MN 55905, USA
* Corresponding author.

Crit Care Nurs Clin N Am 24 (2012) 261–274
doi:10.1016/j.ccell.2012.03.003
0899-5885/12/$ – see front matter © 2012 Elsevier Inc. All rights reserved.

ccnursing.theclinics.com

saline, infections, and snake bites.[5,7–22] Although it is difficult to determine the true incidence of forearm compartment syndrome as well as the mechanisms that are most likely to cause it, many surgeons agree that fractures of the forearm and the distal radius are responsible for a large number of forearm compartment syndromes. In one report it was estimated that 18% of all compartment syndromes, including both upper and lower extremities, are caused by forearm fractures.[4] In analyzing the epidemiology of pediatric forearm compartment syndrome, Grottkau and colleagues[5] used a review of a national trauma database to determine that the incidence of forearm compartment syndromes was just over 1% in the setting of pediatric upper extremity fractures, and more frequent in open fractures than in closed fractures. In an excellent review of compartment syndromes of both the upper and lower extremities, McQueen and colleagues,[6] attempted to quantify the number and incidence of forearm compartment syndromes. This series comprised 164 patients with compartment syndrome of all types. For classification purposes, patients were given the diagnosis of compartment syndrome when the pressure differential between the diastolic blood pressure and that of the affected tissue was less than 30 mm Hg. The second most common fracture in their series was that of the distal radius. Overall, they treated just over 6000 distal radius fractures during the time encompassed by this review, leading them to determine that the incidence of compartment syndrome with distal radius fractures was 0.25%. Also during this time they treated 13 patients with diaphyseal fractures of the forearm who had compartment syndrome. There were a total of 422 patients with this type of fracture, giving an incidence of 3.1% for forearm compartment syndrome in the setting of diaphyseal forearm fracture. The vast majority of patients with upper extremity compartment syndrome in their series were under 35 years of age. Furthermore, the difference in incidence of compartment syndrome in patients under 35 years old and those over 35 years old was significant. Based on their results, they recommended monitoring of forearm compartment pressures in patients who are under 35 years of age, and who have had high-energy fractures of the forearm diaphysis or distal radius.

PATHOPHYSIOLOGY

The most popular theory regarding the pathophysiology of compartment syndrome, including that of the forearm, is the arteriovenous pressure gradient differential theory.[23–25] This theory postulates that as the compartment pressure rises, intraluminal venous pressure also rises leading to a reduction in the arteriovenous pressure gradient. Because of the lack of musculature in the venule wall media, only a relatively small rise in pressure is required to collapse the venule walls. The diminishment of hydrostatic gradient causes reduced local perfusion. The reduced venous drainage seen with increasing compartment pressure causes a rise in the interstitial pressure with formation of tissue edema. This edema, combined with the collapse of forearm lymphatic vessels as a result of the rising pressure, helps contribute to increasing tissue pressure, thus perpetually repeating the cascade of events described above, at least until decompression is performed (**Fig. 1**).[4]

There have been animal studies that attempt to further clarify the pathophysiology of compartment syndrome. One was that of a mouse model with an induced closed soft tissue injury.[26] This group's analysis of the microcirculation following closed soft tissue injury seems to lend credence to the arteriovenous pressure gradient theory, and they further state that leukocyte endothelial cell interaction contributes to this positive feedback cycle in that intravascular leakage and edema formation further serve to cause tissue damage. Although this experimental method did not induce compartment syndromes per se in the mouse model, the mechanics of the

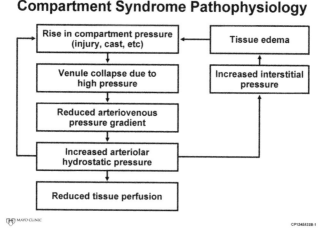

Compartment Syndrome Pathophysiology

Fig. 1. Compartment syndrome cascade of events.

microcirculatory derangement that were demonstrated in this experiment could potentially be extrapolated to help explain the pathophysiology of compartment syndrome in general. In one of the more compelling animal models, Vollmar's group[25] used a hamster striated muscle model to help determine the pathophysiology of compartment syndrome. They found that cessation of blood flow in the aterioles varies with the diameter, specifically that more external pressure is required to stop flow in a larger-diameter vessel. At the same time, it was determined that the venules of all sizes were more prone to collapse with smaller increases in pressure. They demonstrated that the lack of changes in arteriolar diameter, coupled with the easily reduced venular diameter, leads to a reduction in arteriovenous pressure gradient. This group feels that this is the chief mechanism for compression-induced blood flow diminishment. They further state that their findings of a lack of collapse of the arteriolar mechanism and a relative lack of spasm in the arteriolar system negates previous theories of compartment syndrome pathophysiology, including the critical closing theory and the theory of reflex-mediated vascular spasm.

Although the fluid mechanics of compartment syndrome inducement have yet to be fully explained, the end result is tissue ischemia, which in any situation can lead to the depletion of cellular energy stores. This diminishment of energy stores and cessation of energy production lead to increased levels of free radicals and degradative enzymes. This sequence then progresses to myocyte destruction, a further release of these free radicals and degradative enzymes, and the creation of yet another positive feedback cycle with the end result of further tissue destruction.[27]

ANATOMY

There are four compartments of the forearm: dorsal, superficial volar, deep volar, and the mobile wad. The anatomy of the forearm is such that the deeper forearm musculature is, in general, more prone to ischemic and compressive injury because of fascial boundaries that serve to prevent expansion of these muscles. The radius and the ulna are bridged by the very stiff interosseous membrane. Immediately volar to this membrane are the flexor pollicis longus and flexor digitorum profundus muscles. These are the more frequently damaged muscles in end-stage compartment

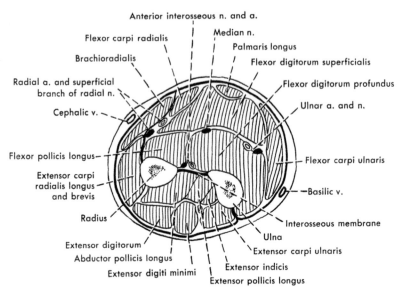

Anterior interosseous n. and a.

Median n.

Flexor carpi radialis

Palmaris longus

Brachioradialis

Flexor digitorum superficialis

Radial a. and superficial
branch of radial n.

Flexor digitorum profundus

Cephalic v.

Ulnar a. and n.

Flexor pollicis longus

Flexor carpi ulnaris

Extensor carpi
radialis longus
and brevis

Basilic v.

Radius

Interosseous membrane

Ulna

Extensor digitorum

Extensor carpi ulnaris

Abductor pollicis longus

Extensor indicis

Extensor digiti minimi

Extensor pollicis longus

Fig. 2. Cross-sectional anatomy of mid-forearm. Note proximity of the flexor pollicis longus and flexor digitorum profundus to the radius, ulna, and interosseus membrane. (*Courtesy of* The Mayo Foundation, Rochester, MN. © Mayo Foundation for Medical Education and Research.)

syndrome (**Fig. 2**). The superficial flexor muscles of the forearm, including the flexor digitorum superficialis, flexor carpi ulnaris, and flexor carpi radialis, are also prone to ischemic injury but appear to be less so because of their more superficial position and somewhat less-stiff superficial fascia. On the dorsum of the forearm are the wrist and finger extensors that again can be damaged with forearm compartment syndrome but not as frequently as those of the deep flexor compartments. Finally, the mobile wad of the forearm consisting of the brachioradialis and the radial wrist extensors can also be damaged in the setting of forearm compartment syndrome. Contractures of the mobile wad are not common, but there is at least one case report of isolated mobile wad ischemic contracture following supracondylar humerus fracture.[8]

Owing to its deeper course in the volar forearm, the median nerve is most frequently damaged with forearm compartment syndrome, and is often encased by fibrosis in the setting of Volkmann's ischemic contracture. In the mid-forearm, the median nerve proper runs between the deep and superficial volar forearm compartments. Additionally, the anterior interosseous nerve (AIN) is found in the floor of the deep volar compartment. The AIN provides motor innervation to the deep flexors (flexor digitorum profundus and flexor pollicis longus), thus a compartment syndrome primarily affecting the deep volar compartment can have a doubly devastating result on these finger flexors. The ulnar nerve can also be affected by compartment syndrome, especially those resulting in a severe ischemic contracture. In the mid-forearm, the ulnar nerve is bounded by the flexor digitorum superficialis, the flexor carpi ulnaris, and the flexor digitorum profundus. Despite being relatively more superficial than the median nerve, the ulnar nerve can certainly suffer significant damage as a result of compartment syndrome. Finally, the radial nerve proper runs in the floor of the mobile wad and the posterior interosseus nerve (PIN) is in the floor of the dorsal compartment. The position of the radial nerve and PIN makes them

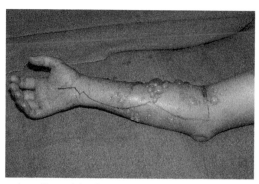

Fig. 3. Upper extremity affected by forearm compartment syndrome. Note the hand in intrinsic-minus position, and the skin changes including cutaneous bullae.

somewhat less prone to ischemic damage; however, they can still be affected by forearm compartment syndrome, especially if severe enough to involve the dorsal forearm or mobile wad.

DIAGNOSIS

In general, the diagnosis of forearm compartment syndrome is a clinical one based on a keen index of suspicion, but is often supplemented by objective diagnostic testing. Traditionally, it has been taught that compartment syndrome will manifest itself with the five "P's": pain, pallor, pulselessness, pain with passive stretch of muscles, and paresthesias. However, *one should note that pulselessness is typically a late or even end-stage finding and does not always accompany compartment syndrome; therefore, one should not dismiss the diagnosis of compartment syndrome when pulses are intact* . Forearm compartment syndromes in general demonstrate a tense swelling of the musculature of the forearm, and in later stages there can even be skin manifestations including epidermolysis and blistering (**Fig. 3**). In a review of the diagnosis of compartment syndrome in obtunded patients, Ouellette[28] justifiably states that most, if not all of the five "P's" can be unreliable in patients with diminished mentation. However, the hand in intrinsic-minus position at rest can be confirmatory for the diagnosis of forearm compartment syndrome. In general, the five "P's" mentioned above are a helpful memory tool to assist with the diagnosis of compartment syndrome; however, one should not wait for all five of these diagnostic criteria to present themselves. If there is suspicion of forearm compartment syndrome one should not hesitate to obtain objective data, which will be discussed in this article, or even to proceed to surgical intervention.

Because forearm compartment syndrome can be easily caused by external compressive forces, a critical step in diagnosis is removal of any dressings that may cause compression of the forearm including plaster or fiberglass casts or splints. Many times this will cause at least partial resolution of the symptoms or findings that the patient manifests. Additionally, internal compression attributable to displaced fracture fragments can be at least partially ameliorated by fracture reduction, especially fractures of the supracondylar humerus and distal radius.

In an effort to supplement clinical findings with objective numerical data, several techniques have been developed to assist with a diagnosis of forearm compartment syndrome. Some of these techniques are well established while others can be considered experimental. Seiler's group[29] attempted to obtain normative data for adult forearms by measuring compartment syndrome pressure. Using 20 volunteers they measured compartment syndrome pressures of the forearm using a commercially available percutaneous fluid transduction pressure. The mean pressure was 9 mm Hg with no significant differences between men and women; dominant and nondominant hands; and position of measurement with regard to proximal, middle, or distal aspect of the forearm. However, there was a slightly higher (albeit statistically insignificant) value in the proximal forearm in this series of patients. The guideline for compartment pressures that are indicative of compartment syndrome are compartment pressure greater than 30 mm Hg and in hypotensive patients, a differential between the diastolic blood pressure and that of the compartment of less than 20 mm Hg. It should be noted, however, that these numerical values are not hard and fast and should be corroborated with clinical examination findings to determine the presence or absence of compartment syndrome and the need for operative decompression.

The initial attempts at objective measurement of compartment pressures were done with a fluid transducer mechanism. The earliest compartment pressure measurement devices were taken with a relatively easy-to-construct apparatus that consisted of a three-way stop cock, one end of which was connected to a needle that was inserted into the compartment. The other end was connected to a manometer and the side of the stop cock was connected to a syringe filled with air. The problems with this mechanism were twofold in that they required injection of a small amount of saline into the compartment and the actual mechanism of the setup was not standardized. Further modifications led to a continuous-infusion pressure transducer **(Fig. 4)**; however, many clinicians were and are hesitant to use this technique as it involves continuous infusion of volume into an already questionable forearm compartment. The chief advantage of the infusion technique is its ability to provide continuous monitoring.[27] A reliable and readily available compartment pressure measurement method is connection of a needle to the arterial pressure monitor, which is easily found in any ICU setting.[28] Some of the more recent advances include the use of the wick catheter or percutaneous needle in the commercialized pressure

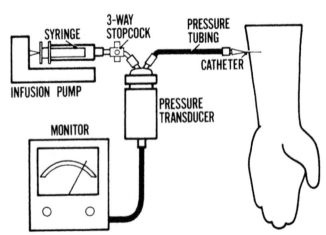

Fig. 4. Diagram of compartment pressure monitor setup using fluid infusion technique. (*From* Gulgonen A. Acute compartment syndrome. In: Green DP, Hotchkiss RN, Pederson WC, et al, editors. Green's Operative Hand Surgery. 5th edition. Philadelphia: Elsevier; 2005. p. 1986–96; with permission.)

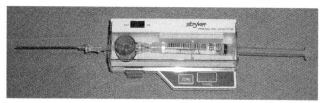

Fig. 5. Commercially available compartment pressure monitor.

transducers that again are fluid based but do not require infusion of fluid into the forearm compartment (**Fig. 5**).[27]

Other groups have attempted to use other diagnostic modalities to provide objective data in the diagnosis of suspected compartment syndrome. Korhonen's group[30] studied the use of electromyography and myotonometry in diagnosing chronic compartment syndrome. It was found that there were correlative changes on these studies seen with an increase in intramuscular pressure but they advised that these tests should not be used alone to diagnose compartment syndrome. While magnetic resonance imaging has been found to be somewhat useful in the determination of the amount of tissue edema within the affected compartment or compartments, it also cannot be used as a primary diagnostic modality.[4,27] Other diagnostic adjuncts that have been used with mixed results include somatosensory evoked potentials, scintigraphy, laser Doppler, and near-infrared spectroscopy; however, none of these have reached mainstream status in the diagnosis of compartment syndrome and at this point can only be considered experimental.[4,27]

NONOPERATIVE TREATMENT

The phrase "nonoperative treatment of compartment syndrome" is a bit of a misnomer because if a patient truly has a forearm compartment syndrome, surgical treatment is a must. There are case reports in the literature that are listed as compartment syndromes, and were successfully treated with observation;[10,16] however, by their own admission, they were "transient," from which one can infer that true ischemia had not occurred. Our own anecdotal experience contains patients who have had mild or moderately tense forearms and borderline compartment pressures for whom we performed serial compartment pressure measurements, and who did not undergo surgery. These patients likely did not have compartment syndrome and were in what could be called a prodromal state before tissue ischemia. One should note that observation of a tense forearm is a tenuous proposition, and if there is any question whatsoever of muscular or neural compromise, decompression should be instituted without delay.

SURGICAL TECHNIQUES

Once the diagnosis of forearm compartment syndrome is made based on clinical exam and objective data, it is of the utmost importance to intervene quickly. Whereas some groups have written about observation of compartment syndrome without surgical decompression it should be noted that these are isolated case reports and there is some question as to whether the diagnosis of forearm compartment syndrome truly applied in these patients' cases.[10,16] If a patient is given the diagnosis of forearm compartment syndrome, the onus is on the treating physician to provide adequate surgical treatment.

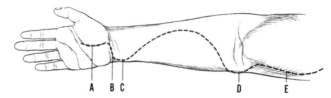

Fig. 6. Common incision pattern for fasciotomy of the volar forearm. (*From* Gulgonen A. Acute compartment syndrome. In: Green DP, Hotchkiss RN, Pederson WC, et al, editors. Green's Operative Hand Surgery. 5th edition. Philadelphia: Elsevier; 2005. p. 1986–96; with permission.)

In general, the decompression of the tense forearm involves performing fasciotomies of both volar forearm compartments as well as the mobile wad and the dorsal compartment of the forearm. Classically, this has been done through two incisions, one on the volar forearm and one on the dorsal forearm (**Fig. 6**). Some groups have noted in cadaveric and dye injection studies that it is possible to adequately decompress both volar and dorsal forearm compartments through solely a volar approach with no incisions on the dorsum of the forearm. However, if one chooses to proceed in this manner, close monitoring of the dorsal forearm compartment is required, both before and after volar decompression.[31–33]

When decompressing the forearm, pneumatic tourniquets are not typically used as the postdecompression perfusion of the forearm musculature must be assessed. The incision on the volar side of the forearm typically begins in the antecubital fossa and extends to the wrist. Some authors have advocated routine decompression of the carpal tunnel in conjunction with forearm fasciotomies as this involves a distal extension of the incision by only a few centimeters.[32] Typically, the incision is carried to the ulnar side of the forearm beginning at the junction of the middle and distal thirds of the forearm, then is curved back to the midline at the level of the carpal tunnel. This then creates a radially based skin flap that will provide coverage of the median nerve within the carpal tunnel, even with large gaping of the wound edges as a result of swelling and edema. Through this volar incision one must access and visualize the muscles of both superficial and deep volar forearm compartments, especially that of the deep compartment, as these muscles, including the flexor pollicis longus and the flexor digitorum profundus, are more prone to ischemic damage based on the architecture of the volar forearm. Once the volar forearm compartments are released close attention should be paid to the musculature of the forearm to ensure reperfusion. If timely intervention has occurred, more often than not these muscles will reperfuse; however, late compartment syndromes may be accompanied by distinctly necrotic muscle that necessitates debridement at the time of fasciotomy. One can easily decompress both the mobile wad and the dorsal forearm compartment through a simple linear incision on the dorsal side of the forearm and the same principles of analysis of muscle perfusion apply.

Some authors have written about the utility of various patterns of incision for forearm fasciotomy, especially on the volar side of the forearm. Gelberman and colleagues[33] used both a curvilinear and a volar ulnar incision in a cadaver study. He stated that both of these incisions provided adequate access to both the superficial and deep volar forearm compartment (**Fig. 7**). Ronel's group[34] performed another cadaver study of approaches to the deep forearm spaces. This group states that their initial motivation for performing the study was that a rational approach to the forearm compartments did not exist, a debatable statement. They assert that, in general, the

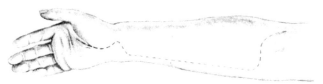

Fig. 7. Variation of incision pattern for volar forearm fasciotomy using an ulnar-sided approach. (*From* Gelberman R, Zakaib GS, Mubarak SJ, et al. Decompression of forearm compartment syndromes. Clin Orthop Rel Research 1978;134:225–9; with permission.)

approach to the volar forearm must provide adequate access to the pronator quadratus, the flexor pollicis longus, and the flexor digitorum profundus. Three approaches to the volar forearm and one on the dorsum were tested. On the volar side, these approaches were deemed "radial," "central," and "ulnar." In terms of injuries to nerves and vascular structures, it was found that the dorsal approach used was perfectly safe. They further stated that the safest approach to both superficial and deep volar forearm compartments was an ulnar-sided one, followed by the central and radial approaches in order of decreasing safety. While these data are valuable, one should not feel constrained by a particular incision pattern and should use an approach to the volar forearm that provides the practitioner with the greatest comfort as well as adequate access to all of the volar forearm compartments.

After completing the fasciotomy or fasciotomies, the wounds are left open so as not to recreate any compressive forces with skin closure. Some practitioners will place retention sutures across the wound, or span the wound with a continuous elastic material such as a vessel loop (colloquially know as "Jacob's ladder" or "Roman sandal"), in an effort to retard wound edge retraction. Another common practice is the placement of a negative pressure dressing over the wound. These dressings are beneficial in that the patient has fewer dressing changes to endure, wound edema is evacuated, and some shrinkage of the wound can be seen. The wounds are later addressed with delayed primary closure or split-thickness skin grafting once edema has diminished and the wounds remain clean.

OUTCOMES

Although compartment syndrome of the forearm has the potential for devastating consequences, if intervention is provided on a prompt basis, quite often these patients will recover fully with minimal residual dysfunction of the forearm or hand.[9,11,17,21,32] At this time, there are no prospective studies that demonstrate the amount of recovery that can be expected following decompression. There was, however, a recent study attempting to correlate outcome with time elapsed from diagnosis to fasciotomy.[35] No clear difference was shown, specifically, short intervals from diagnosis to fasciotomy could result in residual dysfunction while comparatively longer intervals had near-normal outcomes.

Unfortunately there are times, even when intervention is provided on an expeditious basis, that patients do have residual dysfunction. While a forearm contracture attributable to compartment syndrome has traditionally been called a Volkmann's ischemia contracture, there is, in reality, a continuum of dysfunction seen with this problem ranging from mild dysfunction to near total disability of the affected forearm and hand. In an illustration of the marked differences in early and late intervention with forearm compartment syndrome, Ragland's group[36] describes their experience with the quite rare problem of neonatal forearm compartment syndrome. Within their series

Table 1
Classification scheme for Volkmann's ischemic contracture

Type	Flexor Findings	Extensor Findings	Neurologic Findings	Other Findings
1 (Mild)	Partial FDP	None	None to minimal	None
2 (Moderate)	FDP and FPL; variable FDS, FCU, FCR	None to minimal	Present (median > ulnar)	None
3 (Severe)	All flexors	Variable	Severe median and ulnar	Joint contractures, bone deformities, skin scarring

Abbreviations: FCR, flexor carpi radialis; FCU, flexor carpi ulnaris; FDP, flexor digitorum profundus; FDS, flexor digitorum superficialis; FPL, flexor pollicis longus.

Adapted from Tsuge K. Treatment of established Volkmann's contracture. J Bone Joint Surg 1975;57(7):925–9.

of 24 patients, only 1 patient was seen within 24 hours of birth, and that patient underwent forearm fasciotomies very quickly following diagnosis. That particular patient had a good outcome with no residual dysfunction. Unfortunately, the remaining 23 patients in this series were not recognized as having forearm compartment syndrome until much later and all 23 had residual dysfunction of the hand and forearm, at times quite severe. Fifteen required surgical reconstructive procedures for their Volkmann's contracture and several of these patients underwent multiple procedures. In some ways this study illustrates the benefit of prompt recognition of the problem of forearm compartment syndrome combined with early surgical intervention.

VOLKMANN'S ISCHEMIC CONTRACTURE

The most widely used classification of ischemic contracture of the forearm was provided by Tsuge (**Table 1**).[1] This is a three-part classification scheme in which class 1 is mild ischemic contracture affecting mainly the flexor digitorum profundus (FDP). Class 2 affects the FDP as well as the flexor pollicis longus, pronator teres, and to some degree the flexor digitorum superficialis and flexor carpi ulnaris. The most severe class of injury within Tsuge's classification is class 3, which included ischemic damage to essentially all of the flexors in the forearm as well as some damage to the structures of the mobile wad and the dorsal forearm compartment. In reality, as stated earlier, the damage seen in late-stage compartment syndrome is a continuum that ranges from mild damage and dysfunction up to devastating ischemia and necrosis of the forearm musculature. The treatment of Volkmann's ischemic contracture, like treatment of any other upper extremity problem, aims to help correct dysfunction of the upper extremity. While the reconstructive techniques that are used for Volkmann's ischemic contracture can greatly improve the function of the affected upper extremity, eventual normal-functioning of the affected limb should not be expected. The general principles of reconstruction of the forearm affected by Volkmann's ischemic contracture include exposure of the forearm musculature, debridement of any fibrotic and nonfunctioning muscle, and neurolysis, especially that of the median and ulnar nerves. Once excision and neurolysis have been performed, there are a variety of techniques that can be used to help improve function of the forearm. For mild contractures, the flexor/pronator slide can be used to improve the position of the hand as well as function of the forearm flexors. Obviously, a prerequisite for this

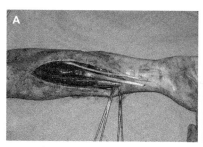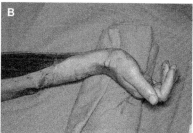

Fig. 8. (*A, B*) Tendon transfers to restore function following extensor muscle damage attributable to compartment syndrome. The palmaris longus is transferred to the extensor pollicis longus, and the flexor digitorum superficialis of the ring finger is transferred to the extensor digitorum communis.

procedure is residual function of the forearm flexors in the setting of mild shortening. This procedure involves detachment of the flexor pronator aponeurosis from the proximal forearm and a distally directed slide, followed by suture pexy of the musculature. By moving the origin distally, the flexion contracture is relieved, thereby allowing for improved function of the hand.[37] In the forearm contractures that are classified as moderate or Class 2, several groups have written about both tendon lengthening and tendon transposition. These have been met with somewhat mixed results especially that of tendon lengthening. The problem with tendon lengthening is recurrence because of scar contracture, which is the chief reason for this procedure's mixed results.[38,39] Tendon transfer can be used for moderate contractures where a specific dysfunction occurs. This transfer is most commonly performed with an extensor tendon, although flexor tendons can be used in the case of dorsal muscle necrosis (**Fig. 8**A, B).[27,38] At this time, the current standard of treatment for severe, grade 3 Volkmann's ischemic contracture is free muscle transfer. This is most frequently performed using a gracilis muscle, and neurotizing it via its branch from the obturator nerve.[2,27,40] The advantage of transfer of a free-functioning muscle is that it imports tissue that has been entirely unaffected by the ischemic insult that initially compromised the forearm. The chief drawback is that it does require microsurgical expertise as well as a sometimes lengthy interval of time for reinnervation of the transferred muscle.

CHRONIC COMPARTMENT SYNDROME

When discussing forearm compartment syndrome, one must mention the entity that has been deemed chronic compartment syndrome. Although this problem does not share the same pathophysiology as does that of acute compartment syndrome, some of the same principles of diagnosis and treatment apply. It is generally agreed that chronic compartment syndrome is an effect of exertion of the forearm musculature and is commonly seen in persons who perform high-impact exercise or work activities.[3,41,42] One case report of two patients with chronic compartment syndrome mentions the use of compartment monitoring via pressure transducer to help assist in the diagnosis.[42] This group found, at times, enormous pressures of the volar forearm compartment with exertion.

As stated earlier, the common denominator between acute compartment syndrome and chronic compartment syndrome is the treatment. In general, only the flexor side of the forearm requires decompression for chronic compartment syndrome and the current literature that exists demonstrates good outcome with volar forearm fasciotomies of varying designs.[3,42]

SUMMARY

Forearm compartment syndrome is a potentially calamitous problem that can befall persons with either injuries or external compression of the forearm. The absolute necessities for a good outcome are early suspicion of forearm compartment syndrome and expeditious surgical intervention. One must be acutely aware of the prospect of compartment syndrome in the settings of forearm diaphysis and distal radius fractures. If forearm fasciotomies are provided to the patient in a rapid fashion, one can expect that most of the time the outcome in terms of the patient's forearm and hand function will be good; however, delays in diagnosis and surgical intervention can lead to ischemic contracture of the forearm that can be manifested in varying degrees but ultimately can lead to greatly diminished function of the affected upper extremity. When a Volkmann's ischemic contracture has occurred, there are surgical interventions to help improve the function of the affected upper extremity but these techniques are in no way a substitute for prompt diagnosis and treatment of acute compartment syndromes.

REFERENCES

1. Tsuge K. Treatment of established Volkmann's contracture. J Bone Joint Surg Am 1975;57(7):925–9.
2. Stevanovic M, Sharpe F. Management of established Volkmann's contracture of the forearm in children. Hand Clin 2006;22(1):99–111.
3. Zandi H, Bell S. Results of compartment decompression in chronic forearm compartment syndrome: six case presentations. Br J Sports Med 2005;39(9):e35, 1–4.
4. Elliott KG, Johnstone AJ. Diagnosing acute compartment syndrome. J Bone Joint Surg Br 2003;85(5):625–32.
5. Grottkau BE, Epps HR, Di Scala C. Compartment syndrome in children and adolescents. J Pediatr Surg 2005;40(4):678–82.
6. McQueen MM, Gaston P, Court-Brown CM. Acute compartment syndrome. Who is at risk?. J Bone Joint Surg Br 2000;82(2):200–3.
7. Ananthanarayan C, Castro C, McKee N, et al. Compartment syndrome following intravenous regional anesthesia. Can J Anaesth 2000;47(11):1094–8.
8. Baek GH, Kim JS, Chung MS. Isolated ischemic contracture of the mobile wad: a report of two cases. J Hand Surg [Br] 2004;29(5):508–9.
9. Baeten Y, De Smet L, Fabry G. Acute anterior forearm compartment syndrome following wrist arthrodesis. Acta Orthop Belg 1999;65(2):239–41.
10. Cohen J, Bush S. Case report: compartment syndrome after a suspected black widow spider bite. Ann Emerg Med 2005;45(4):414–6.
11. Cosker T, Gupta S, Tayton K. Compartment syndrome caused by suction. Injury 2004;35(11):1194–5.
12. Docker C, Titley OG. A case of forearm compartment syndrome following a ring avulsion injury. Injury 2002;33(3):274–5.
13. Edwards JJ, Samuels D, Fu ES. Forearm compartment syndrome from intravenous mannitol extravasation during general anesthesia. Anesth Analg 2003;96(1):245–6.
14. Funk L, Grover D, de Silva H. Compartment syndrome of the hand following intra-arterial injection of heroin. J Hand Surg [Br] 1999;24(3):366–7.
15. Namboothiri S. Compartment syndrome and systemic hypertension. J Bone Joint Surg Br 2005;87(10):1420–2.

16. O'Neil D, Sheppard JE. Transient compartment syndrome of the forearm resulting from venous congestion from a tourniquet. J Hand Surg [Am] 1989;14(5):894–6.

17. Quigley JT, Popich GA, Lanz UB. Compartment syndrome of the forearm and hand: a case report. Clin Orthop Relat Res 1981;161:247–51.

18. Roberts RS, Csencsitz TA, Heard CW Jr. Upper extremity compartment syndromes following pit viper envenomation. Clin Orthop Relat Res 1985;193:184–8.

19. Schnall SB, Holtom PD, Silva E. Compartment syndrome associated with infection of the upper extremity. Clin Orthop Relat Res 1994;306:128–31.

20. Summerfield SL, Folberg CR, Weiss AP. Compartment syndrome of the pronator quadratus: a case report. J Hand Surg [Am] 1997;22(2):266–8.

21. Vaienti L, Vourtsis S, Urzola V. Compartment syndrome of the forearm following an electromyographic assessment. J Hand Surg [Br] 2005;30(6):656–7.

22. Yip TR, Demaerschalk BM. Forearm compartment syndrome following intravenous thrombolytic therapy for acute ischemic stroke. Neurocrit Care 2005;2(1):47–8.

23. Hargens AR, Mubarak SJ. Current concepts in the pathophysiology, evaluation, and diagnosis of compartment syndrome. Hand Clin 1998;14(3):371–83.

24. Mubarak SJ, Hargens AR. Acute compartment syndromes. Surg Clin North Am 1983;63(3):539–65.

25. Vollmar B, Westermann S, Menger MD. Microvascular response to compartment syndrome-like external pressure elevation: an in vivo fluorescence microscopic study in the hamster striated muscle. J Trauma 1999;46(1):91–6.

26. Schaser KD, Vollmar B, Menger MD, et al. In vivo analysis of microcirculation following closed soft-tissue injury. J Orthop Res 1999;17(5):678–85.

27. Gulgonen A. Acute compartment syndrome. In: Green DP, Hotchkiss RN, Pederson WC, et al, editors. Green's operative hand surgery. 5th edition. Philadelphia: Elsevier; 2005. p. 1986–96.

28. Ouellette EA. Compartment syndromes in obtunded patients. Hand Clin 1998;14(3):431–50.

29. Seiler JG 3rd, Womack S, De L'Aune WR, et al. Intracompartmental pressure measurements in the normal forearm. J Orthop Trauma 1993;7(5):414–6.

30. Korhonen RK, Vain A, Vanninen E, et al. Can mechanical myotonometry or electromyography be used for the prediction of intramuscular pressure? Physiol Meas 2005;26(6):951–63.

31. Frober R, Linss W. Anatomic bases of the forearm compartment syndrome. Surg Radiol Anat 1994;16(4):341–7.

32. Gelberman RH, Garfin SR, Hergenroeder PT, et al. Compartment syndromes of the forearm: diagnosis and treatment. Clin Orthop Relat Res 1981;161:252–61.

33. Gelberman RH, Zakaib GS, Mubarak SJ, et al. Decompression of forearm compartment syndromes. Clin Orthop Relat Res 1978;134:225–9.

34. Ronel DN, Mtui E, Nolan WB 3rd. Forearm compartment syndrome: anatomical analysis of surgical approaches to the deep space. Plast Reconstr Surg 2004;114(3):697–705.

35. Cascio BM, Pateder DB, Wilckens JH, et al. Compartment syndrome: time from diagnosis to fasciotomy. J Surg Orthop Adv 2005;14(3):117–21.

36. Ragland R 3rd, Moukoko D, Ezaki M, et al. Forearm compartment syndrome in the newborn: report of 24 cases. J Hand Surg [Am] 2005;30(5):997–1003.

37. Eichler GR, Lipscomb PR. The changing treatment of Volkmann's ischemic contractures from 1955 to 1965 at the Mayo Clinic. Clin Orthop Relat Res 1967;50:215–23.

38. Ultee J, Hovius SE. Functional results after treatment of Volkmann's ischemic contracture: a long-term followup study. Clin Orthop Relat Res 2005;431:42–9.

39. Reigstad A, Hellum C. Volkmann's ischaemic contracture of the forearm. Injury 1980;12(2):148–50.
40. Zuker RM. Volkmann's ischemic contracture. Clin Plast Surg 1989;16(3):537–45.
41. Goubier JN, Saillant G. Chronic compartment syndrome of the forearm in competitive motor cyclists: a report of two cases. Br J Sports Med 2003;37(5):452–3 [discussion: 453–4].
42. Soderberg TA. Bilateral chronic compartment syndrome in the forearm and the hand. J Bone Joint Surg Br 1996;78(5):780–2.

Intra-Abdominal Hypertension:
Evolving Concepts

Manu L.N.G. Malbrain, MD, PhD*, Inneke E. De laet, MD

KEYWORDS

- Abdominal pressure • Abdominal hypertension • Abdominal compartment syndrome
- Measurement • Diagnosis • Pathophysiology • Organ support • Treatment

KEY POINTS

- ACS is the end stage of the physiologic sequellae of increased IAP, termed IAH. Recent observations suggest an increasing frequency of this complication in all types of patients.
- In analogy to AKI and ALI, there is certainly a need for basic research into the underlying mechanisms of the new concepts of acute bowel injury and the polycompartment syndrome.
- Currently no good multicentric randomized interventional controlled clinical trial has tackled the question of whether an increase of IAP is a phenomenon or an epiphenomenon and whether any intervention to normalize IAP or APP will eventually affect patient outcome.

A compartment syndrome (CS) exists when increased pressure in a closed anatomic space threatens the viability of enclosed tissue.[1] Within the body there are four types of compartments, the head, the chest, the abdomen, and the extremities, but when a compartment syndrome occurs in the abdominal cavity the impact on end-organ function both within and outside of the cavity can be devastating (**Table 1**). Intra-abdominal hypertension (IAH) is a graded phenomenon and can evolve to the end-stage abdominal compartment syndrome (ACS), which is an all or nothing phenomenon. The ACS is not a disease and as such it can have many causes and it can develop within many disease processes. The development of IAH is of extreme importance in the care of critically ill patients, because of the impact of increased intra-abdominal pressure (IAP) on end-organ function. Recent animal and human data suggest that the adverse effects of elevated IAP can occur at much lower levels than previously thought and even before the development of clinically overt ACS. This

A version of this article was previously published in *Chest Medicine Clinics* 30:1.
Intensive Care Unit, ZiekenhuisNetwerk Antwerpen, Campus Stuivenberg, Lange Beeldekensstraat 267, B-2060 Antwerpen 6, Belgium
* Corresponding author.
E-mail address: manu.malbrain@skynet.be

Crit Care Nurs Clin N Am 24 (2012) 275–309
doi:10.1016/j.ccell.2012.03.004
0899-5885/12/$ – see front matter © 2012 Elsevier Inc. All rights reserved.

ccnursing.theclinics.com

Table 1
The four compartments

	Head	Chest	Abdomen	Extremities
Syndrome	Cerebral herniation	Thoracic compartment syndrome	Abdominal compartment syndrome	Extremity compartment syndrome
Potential implication	Brain death	Cardiopulmonary collapse	Multiple organ dysfunction	Extremity loss
Primary physiologic parameter	Intracranial pressure (ICP)	Intrathoracic pressure (ITP)	Intra-abdominal pressure (IAP)	Extremity compartment pressures (CP)
Secondary parameter	Cerebral perfusion pressure (CPP)	Peak/mean airway pressure	Abdominal perfusion pressure (APP)	Peripheral arterial perfusion pressure
Fluid	Cerebrospinal fluid (CSF)	Pleural fluid	Ascites	Interstitial fluid
Enclosure	Skull	Rib cage	Abdominal cage	Muscle fascia
Therapeutic intervention	Lower ICP: CSF drainage Increase CPP: vasopressors, fluids	Lower ITP Escharotomy, chest tube	Lower IAP: ascites drainage Increase APP: vasopressors, fluids	Lower CP
Resuscitative plan	Open compartment Decompressive craniectomy	Open compartment Decompressive sternotomy	Open compartment Decompressive laparotomy	Open compartment Decompressive fasciotomy
Importance	Adaptation of ventilatory support essential	Recognition of syndrome can be life saving	Prevention of bacterial translocation and MODS can be life saving	Recognition can be limb saving

Abbreviations: APP, abdominal perfusion pressure; CP, compartment pressure; CPP, cerebral perfusion pressure; CSF, cerebrospinal fluid; IAP, intra-abdominal pressure; ICP, intracranial pressure; ITP, intrathoracic pressure; MODS, multiple organ dysfunction syndrome.
Adapted from Cheatham M. Compartment syndrome. The four compartment syndromes. 2008. Available at: http://www.surgicalcriticalcare.net/Lectures/compartment_syndrome.pdf; with permission.

review gives a concise overview of the definitions, epidemiology, pathophysiology, and management of IAH and ACS.

DEFINITIONS

The term ACS was first used by Fietsam and colleagues[2] in the late 1980s to describe the pathophysiologic alterations resulting from IAH secondary to aortic aneurysm surgery: "In four patients that received more than 25 L of fluid resuscitation increased IAP developed after aneurysm repair. It was manifested by increased ventilatory pressure, increased central venous pressure, and decreased urinary output. This set of findings constitutes an *abdominal compartment syndrome* caused by massive interstitial and retroperitoneal swelling... Opening the abdominal incision was associated with dramatic improvements ...."

The World Society on Abdominal Compartment Syndrome (WSACS, www.wsacs. org) was founded in 2004 to serve as a peer-reviewed forum and educational resource for all health care providers as well as industry who have an interest in IAH and ACS. Recently the first consensus definitions on IAH and ACS have been published.[1,3] **Table 2** summarizes these consensus definitions: a sustained increase in IAP equal to or above 12 mm Hg defines IAH where ACS is defined by a sustained IAP above 20 mm Hg with new-onset or progressive organ failure.

RECOGNITION OF ABDOMINAL COMPARTMENT SYNDROME
Clinical Awareness

Despite an escalation of the medical literature on the subject, there still appears to be an underrecognition of the syndrome. The results of several surveys on the physician's knowledge of IAH and ACS have recently been published.[4,5] The bottom line is that there is still a general lack of clinical awareness and many ICUs never measure the IAP. No consensus exists on optimal timing of measurement or decompression. In a recent editorial, Ivatury[6] states that: "One potential exegesis of this widespread under-appreciation of these syndromes may be related to our rapidly evolving understanding of their patho-physiology. Our knowledge is no longer restricted to experimentally sound (isolated IAH) concepts, but is elevated to a true clinical phenomenon (IAH as a 'second-hit' after ischemia-reperfusion)."

Etiology

The ACS can be diagnosed when there is increased IAP with evidence of end-organ dysfunction. Although multiple causes of acute cardiopulmonary, renal, hepatosplanchnic, or neurologic deterioration exist in the ICU, it is important that we recognize IAP as being an independent risk factor for this organ function deterioration. Hence, the timely recognition of the underlying risk factors and predisposing conditions that lead to IAH and ACS is extremely important. Indications for IAP monitoring should be based on the presence/absence of these risk factors. Many conditions are reported in association with IAH/ACS, and they can be classified into four categories: first, conditions that decrease abdominal wall compliance; second, conditions that increase intraluminal contents; third, conditions related to abdominal collections of fluid, air, or blood; and finally, conditions related to capillary leak and fluid resuscitation. **Box 1** lists some of the clinical conditions related to these four categories.

Hence, it becomes clear that ACS can develop both in nonsurgical and surgical patients. An algorithm for the assessment of IAH is proposed in **Fig. 1**.

Table 2
Consensus definitions

Definition 1	IAP is the steady-state pressure concealed within the abdominal cavity.
Definition 2	APP = MAP − IAP
Definition 3	FG = GFP − PTP = MAP − 2 * IAP
Definition 4	IAP should be expressed in mm Hg and measured at end-expiration in the complete supine position after ensuring that abdominal muscle contractions are absent and with the transducer zeroed at the level of the mid-axillary line.
Definition 5	The reference standard for intermittent IAP measurement is via the bladder with a maximal instillation volume of 25 mL of sterile saline.
Definition 6	Normal IAP is approximately 5–7 mm Hg in critically ill adults.
Definition 7	IAH is defined by a sustained or repeated pathologic elevation of IAP ≥ 12 mmHg.
Definition 8	IAH is graded as follows: Grade I: IAP 12–15 mm Hg Grade II: IAP 16–20 mm Hg Grade III: IAP 21–25 mm Hg Grade IV: IAP >25 mm Hg
Definition 9	ACS is defined as a sustained IAP >20 mm Hg (with or without an APP <60 mm Hg) that is associated with new organ dysfunction/failure.
Definition 10	Primary ACS is a condition associated with injury or disease in the abdomino-pelvic region that frequently requires early surgical or interventional radiological intervention.
Definition 11	Secondary ACS refers to conditions that do not originate from the abdomino-pelvic region.
Definition 12	Recurrent ACS refers to the condition in which ACS redevelops following previous surgical or medical treatment of primary or secondary ACS.

Abbreviations: ACS, abdominal compartment syndrome; APP, abdominal perfusion pressure; FG, filtration gradient; GFP, glomerular filtration pressure; IAH, intra-abdominal hypertension; IAP, intra-abdominal pressure; MAP, mean arterial pressure; PTP, proximal tubular pressure.

Adapted from Malbrain ML, Cheatham ML, Kirkpatrick A, et al. Results from the International Conference of Experts on Intra-abdominal Hypertension and Abdominal Compartment Syndrome. I. Definitions. Intensive Care Med 2006;32:1722–32; with permission.

DIAGNOSIS
Clinical and Radiologic Examination

The abdominal perimeter or girth cannot be used as a surrogate for IAP because it only poorly correlates with it. Studies have shown that clinical IAP estimation is also far from accurate with a sensitivity and positive predictive value of around 40% to 60%.[7,8] Radiologic investigation with plain radiography of the chest or abdomen, abdominal ultrasound, or CT scan is also insensitive to the presence of increased IAP.

Measurement of Intra-Abdominal Pressure

Because the abdomen and its contents can be considered as relatively noncompressive and primarily fluid in character, behaving in accordance with Pascal's law, the IAP measured at one point may be assumed to represent the IAP throughout the abdomen.[9,10] The IAP is therefore defined as the steady-state pressure concealed within the abdominal cavity, IAP increases with inspiration (diaphragmatic contraction) and decreases with expiration (diaphragmatic relaxation).

Box 1

Risk factors for the development of IAH and ACS

Related to diminished abdominal wall compliance

- Mechanical ventilation, especially fighting with the ventilator and the use of accessory muscles
- Use of positive end expiratory pressure (PEEP) or the presence of auto-PEEP
- Basal pneumonia
- High body mass index
- Pneumoperitoneum
- Abdominal (vascular) surgery, especially with tight abdominal closures
- Pneumatic anti-shock garments
- Prone and other body positioning
- Abdominal wall bleeding or rectus sheath hematomas
- Correction of large hernias, gastroschisis, or omphalocele
- Burns with abdominal eschars

Related to increased intra-abdominal contents

- Gastroparesis
- Gastric distention
- Ileus
- Volvulus
- Colonic pseudo-obstruction
- Abdominal tumor
- Retroperitoneal/abdominal wall hematoma
- Enteral feeding
- Intra-abdominal or retroperitoneal tumor
- Damage control laparotomy

Related to abdominal collections of fluid, air, or blood

- Liver dysfunction with ascites
- Abdominal infection (eg, pancreatitis, peritonitis, abscess)
- Hemoperitoneum
- Pneumoperitoneum
- Laparoscopy with excessive inflation pressures
- Major trauma
- Peritoneal dialysis

Related to capillary leak and fluid resuscitation

- Acidosis[a] (pH below 7.2)
- Hypothermia[a] (core temperature below 33°C)
- Coagulopathy[a] (platelet count below 50,000/mm^3 OR an activated partial thromboplastin time [APTT] more than 2 times normal OR a prothrombin time [PTT] below 50% OR an international standardized ratio [INR] more than 1.5)
- Polytransfusion/trauma (>10 units of packed red cells/24 h)
- Sepsis (as defined by the American–European Consensus Conference definitions)
- Severe sepsis or bacteremia
- Septic shock
- Massive fluid resuscitation (>5 L of colloid or >10 L of crystalloid/24 h with capillary leak and positive fluid balance)
- Major burns

[a]The combination of acidosis, hypothermia, and coagulopathy has been described in the literature as the deadly triad.[186,187]

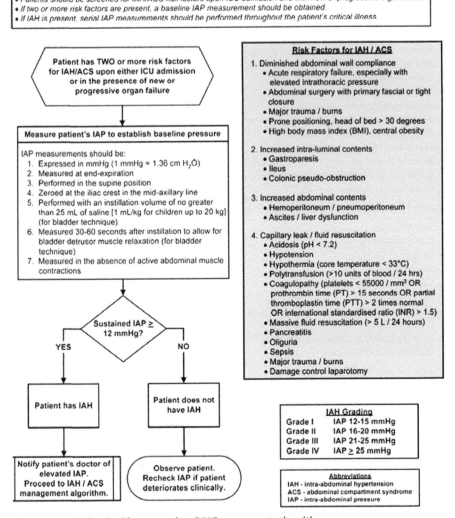

Fig. 1. Intra-abdominal hypertension (IAH) assessment algorithm.

In the strictest sense, normal IAP ranges from 0 to 5 mm Hg.[11] Certain physiologic conditions, however, such as morbid obesity,[12,13] ovarian tumors, cirrhosis, or pregnancy, may be associated with chronic IAP elevations of 10 to 15 mm Hg to which the patient has adapted with an absence of significant pathophysiology. In contrast, children commonly demonstrate low IAP values.[14] The clinical importance of any IAP must be assessed in view of the baseline steady-state IAP for the individual patient.

The key to recognizing ACS in a critically ill patient is the demonstration of elevated IAP: "measuring is knowing!"[15] IAP can be directly measured with an intraperitoneal catheter attached to a pressure transducer. During CO_2-insufflation in laparoscopic surgery IAP is measured directly via the Verres needle.

Different indirect methods for estimating IAP are used clinically because direct measurements are considered to be too invasive.[9,16] These techniques include rectal, uteral, gastric, inferior vena caval, and urinary bladder pressure measurement. Only gastric and bladder pressures are used clinically. Over the years, bladder pressure has been forwarded as the gold-standard indirect method. The bladder technique has achieved the most widespread adoption worldwide because of its simplicity and minimal cost.[9,10] However, considerable variation is noted between the different techniques used, and recent data suggest to instill minimal volumes (10–25 mL) into the bladder for priming.[17–20]

Recently, new measurement kits, either via a FoleyManometer (Holtech Medical, Copenhagen, Denmark, at www.holtech-medical.com), Abdo Pressure (Unomedical, Birkersd, Denmark, at www.unomedical.com) or an AbViser-valve (Wolfe Tory Medical, Salt Lake City, UT, USA, at www.wolfetory.com) have become commercially available.

Continuous Intra-Abdominal Pressure Measurement

The IAP can also be measured via a balloon-tipped stomach catheter (Spiegelberg, Hamburg, Germany, at www.spiegelberg.de and Pulsion Medical Systems, Munich, Germany, at www.pulsion.com).[10] This avoids the problems associated with the creation of a hydrostatic fluid column and allows continuous IAP and APP measurement.[21]

Several other methods for continuous IAP measurement via the stomach, peritoneal cavity (using air-chamber or piezoresistive membranes), and bladder have been validated.[16,22–24] Although these techniques seem promising, further clinical validation needs to be done before their general use can be recommended.

Which Patient?

Although the prevalence and incidence of IAH in critically ill patients is considerable,[25,26] routine IAP measurement in all patients admitted to the ICU is currently rarely performed, and probably not indicated. The ACS can be diagnosed when there is increased IAP with evidence of end-organ dysfunction. While multiple causes of acute cardiopulmonary, renal, hepatosplanchnic, or neurologic deterioration exist in the ICU, it is important that we recognize the IAP as being an independent risk factor for this organ function deterioration. The WSACS has provided a list with risk factors associated with IAH and ACS and if two or more risk factors are present, baseline routine IAP monitoring is advised (**Box 1**).[3,27] Massive volume resuscitation after a "first hit" for any reason (eg, burns, trauma, pancreatitis, hemorrhagic shock) can lead to increased IAP, particularly postoperatively or in a septic patient. The "second hit" probably results from the effects of "capillary leak," shock with ischemia-reperfusion injury and the release of cytokines combined with massive increases in total extracellular volume.[15]

What Technique?

According to the WSACS consensus guidelines, IAP should be measured at end-expiration in the complete supine position after ensuring that abdominal muscle contractions are absent and with the transducer zeroed at the level of the midaxillary line at the iliac crest after an instillation volume of maximal 20 to 25 mL.[1] An intermittent technique may be used for screening, whereas in some patients, a continuous technique may be preferable, eg, when the APP is used as a resuscitation end point, or in patients with impending ACS requiring urgent abdominal decompression.

What Frequency?

When an intermittent method is used, measurements should be obtained at least every 4 to 6 hours, and in patients with evolving organ dysfunction, this frequency should be increased up to hourly measurements.

When to Stop Intra-Abdominal Pressure Measurement?

IAP measurement can be discontinued when the risk factors for IAH are resolved or the patient has no signs of acute organ dysfunction, and IAP values have been below 10 to 12 mm Hg for 24 to 48 hours. In case of recurrent organ dysfunction, IAP measurement should be reconsidered.

What About Intra-Abdominal Pressure Measurement in Children?

Some studies have been performed regarding IAP measurement in children.[14,28] The transvesical route can be used safely in children, but obviously, the instillation volume is important in this population. Davis and colleagues[14] found that 1 mL/kg produces reliable IAP values when compared with higher volumes. Normal IAP values are lower in children up to 40 kg body weight (3–5 mm Hg) and the thresholds defining IAH (9 mm Hg) and ACS (16 mm Hg) are also lower compared with adults.

What About Intra-Abdominal Pressure Measurement in Awake Patients?

IAP measurement is most often performed in sedated patients, where muscle contractions are absent. When measuring IAP in awake patients, specific attention should be made that no muscle contractions are present, eg, during forced expiration in a patient who has chronic obstructive pulmonary disease with auto-PEEP. Adequate pain medication should be administered, especially after abdominal surgery, as even putting the patient in supine position may induce abdominal pain and muscle contractions, leading to elevated IAP readings.

PATHOPHYSIOLOGIC IMPLICATIONS

IAH affects multiple organ systems in a graded fashion. To better understand the clinical presentation and management of disorders of IAH, one must understand the physiologic derangements within each organ system separately.[15] It is beyond the scope of this review to give a concise and complete review of the pathophysiologic implications of raised IAP on end-organ function within and outside the abdominal cavity.[29,30] We will discuss only some key messages related to each organ that will affect daily clinical practice; these are summarized in **Fig. 2**.

Neurologic Function

Acute IAH may cause an increase in intracranial pressure (ICP) because of augmentation in pleural pressure. Cerebral perfusion pressure (CPP) will decrease owing to a functional obstruction of cerebral venous outflow caused by the increased intrathoracic pressure (ITP) owing to the cephalad displacement of the diaphragm in combination with a reduced systemic blood pressure as a result of decreased preload and cardiac output (CO). Cerebral blood flow and jugular bulb saturation will decrease. The effects of IAP on the central nervous system (CNS) have not been extensively studied to date, and remain a challenging area for laboratory and clinical investigators.[31–38]

- Because of the interactions between IAP, ITP, and ICP, accurate monitoring of IAP in head trauma victims with associated abdominal lesions is worthwhile.
- The presence of increased IAP can be an additional "extracranial" cause of intracranial hypertension in patients with abdominal trauma without overt craniocerebral lesions.

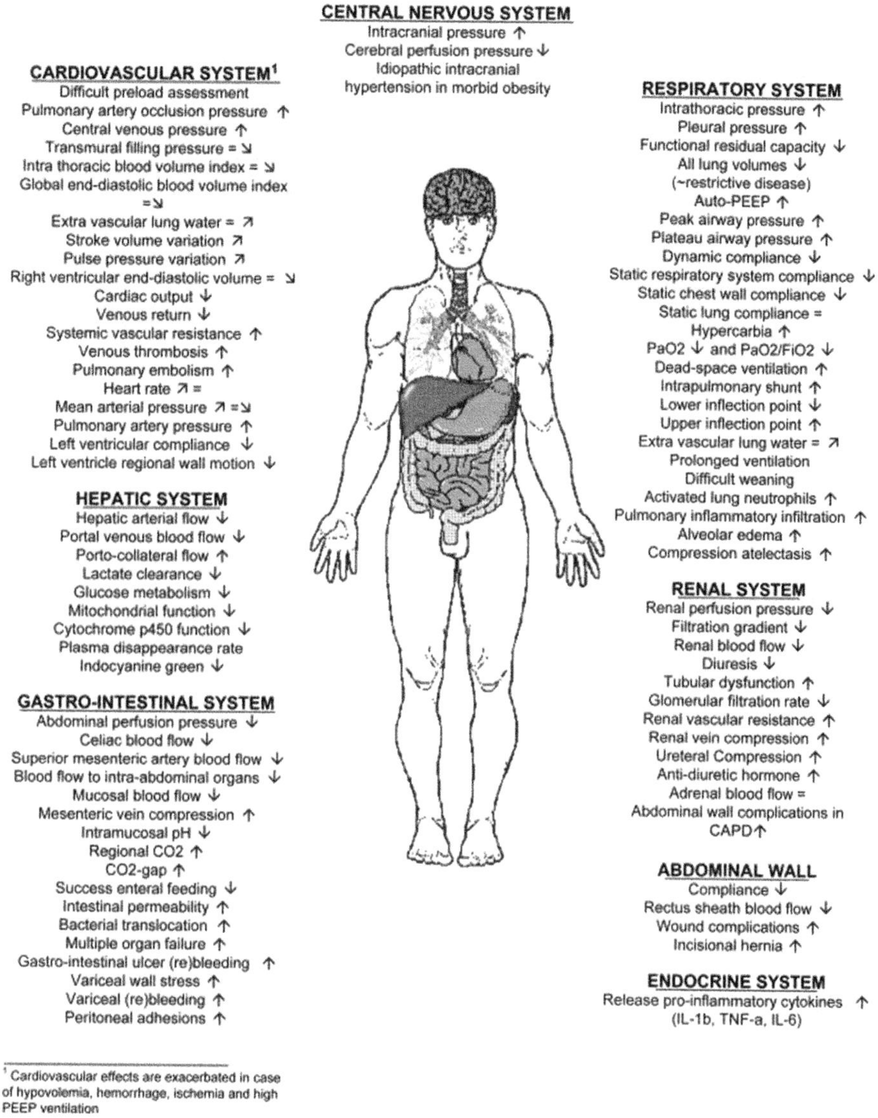

CENTRAL NERVOUS SYSTEM
Intracranial pressure ↑
Cerebral perfusion pressure ↓
Idiopathic intracranial
hypertension in morbid obesity

CARDIOVASCULAR SYSTEM[1]
Difficult preload assessment
Pulmonary artery occlusion pressure ↑
Central venous pressure ↑
Transmural filling pressure = ↘
Intra thoracic blood volume index = ↘
Global end-diastolic blood volume index
= ↘
Extra vascular lung water = ↗
Stroke volume variation ↗
Pulse pressure variation ↗
Right ventricular end-diastolic volume = ↘
Cardiac output ↓
Venous return ↓
Systemic vascular resistance ↑
Venous thrombosis ↑
Pulmonary embolism ↑
Heart rate ↗ =
Mean arterial pressure ↗ =↘
Pulmonary artery pressure ↑
Left ventricular compliance ↓
Left ventricle regional wall motion ↓

HEPATIC SYSTEM
Hepatic arterial flow ↓
Portal venous blood flow ↓
Porto-collateral flow ↑
Lactate clearance ↓
Glucose metabolism ↓
Mitochondrial function ↓
Cytochrome p450 function ↓
Plasma disappearance rate
Indocyanine green ↓

GASTRO-INTESTINAL SYSTEM
Abdominal perfusion pressure ↓
Celiac blood flow ↓
Superior mesenteric artery blood flow ↓
Blood flow to intra-abdominal organs ↓
Mucosal blood flow ↓
Mesenteric vein compression ↑
Intramucosal pH ↓
Regional CO2 ↑
CO2-gap ↑
Success enteral feeding ↓
Intestinal permeability ↑
Bacterial translocation ↑
Multiple organ failure ↑
Gastro-intestinal ulcer (re)bleeding ↑
Variceal wall stress ↑
Variceal (re)bleeding ↑
Peritoneal adhesions ↑

RESPIRATORY SYSTEM
Intrathoracic pressure ↑
Pleural pressure ↑
Functional residual capacity ↓
All lung volumes ↓
(~restrictive disease)
Auto-PEEP ↑
Peak airway pressure ↑
Plateau airway pressure ↑
Dynamic compliance ↓
Static respiratory system compliance ↓
Static chest wall compliance ↓
Static lung compliance =
Hypercarbia ↑
PaO2 ↓ and PaO2/FiO2 ↓
Dead-space ventilation ↑
Intrapulmonary shunt ↑
Lower inflection point ↓
Upper inflection point ↑
Extra vascular lung water = ↗
Prolonged ventilation
Difficult weaning
Activated lung neutrophils ↑
Pulmonary inflammatory infiltration ↑
Alveolar edema ↑
Compression atelectasis ↑

RENAL SYSTEM
Renal perfusion pressure ↓
Filtration gradient ↓
Renal blood flow ↓
Diuresis ↓
Tubular dysfunction ↑
Glomerular filtration rate ↓
Renal vascular resistance ↑
Renal vein compression ↑
Ureteral Compression ↑
Anti-diuretic hormone ↑
Adrenal blood flow =
Abdominal wall complications in
CAPD ↑

ABDOMINAL WALL
Compliance ↓
Rectus sheath blood flow ↓
Wound complications ↑
Incisional hernia ↑

ENDOCRINE SYSTEM
Release pro-inflammatory cytokines ↑
(IL-1b, TNF-a, IL-6)

---

[1] Cardiovascular effects are exacerbated in case of hypovolemia, hemorrhage, ischemia and high PEEP ventilation

Fig. 2. Pathophysiology of intra-abdominal hypertension.

- Laparoscopy in the acute posttraumatic phase is more foe than friend and recent head injury should be considered a contraindication for laparoscopic procedures.[39–41]
- The same principles are responsible for the development of idiopathic intracranial hypertension (pseudotumor cerebri) in morbidly obese patients.[35,42,43]
- Weight loss by bariatric surgery is associated with improvements in ICP and CNS symptoms.[42,44]
- The direct effects of IAH on neurologic function has been ablated by sternotomy, pericardiotomy, or bilateral pleurotomy in experimental conditions.[37]

Cardiovascular Function

Because of the cephalad movement of the diaphragm, pleural pressure and ITP will increase. This will result in a difficult preload assessment because traditional filling pressures will be erroneously increased. When IAP rises above 10 mm Hg, cardiac output (CO) drops because of an increase in afterload and a decrease in preload and left ventricular compliance. Systemic vascular resistance (SVR) increases (owing to mechanical compression of vascular beds) and preload is reduced (owing to drop in stroke volume and a reduction of venous return).[45–48] Mean arterial blood pressure may initially rise as a result of shunting of blood away from the abdominal cavity but thereafter normalizes or decreases.[49,50]

- Cardiovascular dysfunction and failure (low CO, high SVR) are common in IAH or ACS.
- Accurate assessment and optimization of preload, contractility, and afterload is essential to restore end-organ perfusion and function.
- Our understanding of traditional hemodynamic monitoring techniques and parameters, however, must be reevaluated in IAH/ACS, since pressure-based estimates of intravascular volume as pulmonary artery occlusion pressure (PAOP) and central venous pressure (CVP) are erroneously increased.
  - The clinician must be aware of the interactions between ITP, IAP, PEEP, and intracardiac filling pressures.
  - Misinterpretation of the patient's minute-to-minute cardiac status may result in the institution of inappropriate and potentially detrimental therapy.
  - Transmural filling pressures, calculated as the end-expiration value (ee) minus the ITP better reflect preload.[46]
    - CVP = CVPee − ITP
    - PAOP = PAOPee − ITP
  - A quick estimate of transmural filling pressures can also be obtained by subtracting half of the IAP from the end-expiratory filling pressure since abdomino-thoracic pressure transmission has been estimated to be around 50%.
    - CVP = CVPee − IAP/2
    - PAOP = PAOPee − IAP/2
  - The surviving sepsis campaign guidelines targeting initial and ongoing resuscitation toward a CVP of 8 to 12 mm Hg[51] and other studies targeting a MAP of 65 mm Hg[52] should be interpreted with caution in case of IAH/ACS to avoid unnecessary over- and underresuscitation!
- Volumetric estimates of preload status, such as right ventricular end diastolic volume index (RVEDVI) or global end diastolic volume index (GEDVI), are especially useful because of the changing ventricular compliance and elevated ITP.[48,53–56]
- Functional hemodynamic parameters such as stroke volume (SVV) or pulse pressure variation (PPV) but not systolic pressure variation (SPV) should be used to assess volume responsiveness.[57]
- The cardiovascular effects are aggravated by hypovolemia and the application of PEEP,[58–62] whereas hypervolemia has a temporary protective effect.[37]
- Analogous to the widely accepted and clinically used concept of cerebral perfusion pressure, calculated as mean arterial pressure (MAP) minus intracranial pressure (ICP), abdominal perfusion pressure (APP), calculated as MAP minus IAP, has been proposed as a more accurate predictor of visceral perfusion and a potential end point for resuscitation.[33,49,63,64]
  - APP = MAP − IAP

- APP, by considering both arterial inflow (MAP) and restrictions to venous outflow (IAP), has been demonstrated to be statistically superior to either parameter alone in predicting patient survival from IAH and ACS.[49]
- A target APP of at least 60 mm Hg has been demonstrated to correlate with improved survival from IAH and ACS.

Pulmonary Function

The interactions between the abdominal and the thoracic compartment pose a specific challenge to the ICU physicians.[65] Both compartments are linked via the diaphragm and on average a 50% (range 25%–80%) transmission of IAP to the ITP has been noted in previous animal and human studies.[48] Patients with primary ACS will often develop a secondary ARDS and will require a different ventilatory strategy and more specific treatment than a patient with primary ARDS.[66,67] The major problem lies in the reduction of the functional residual capacity (FRC). Together with the alterations caused by secondary ARDS, this will lead to the so-called "baby-lungs." Some key issues to remember are the following:

- IAH decreases total respiratory system compliance by a decrease in chest wall compliance, while lung compliance remains unchanged.[68,69]
- Best PEEP should be set to counteract IAP while in the same time avoiding over-inflation of already well-aerated lung regions.[70]
  - Best PEEP = IAP
- The ARDS consensus definitions should take into account PEEP and IAP values.
- During lung protective ventilation, the plateau pressures should be limited to transmural plateau pressures below 35 cmH_2O.
  - Pplat = Pplat − IAP/2
- The PAOP criterion in ARDS consensus definitions is futile in the case of IAH and should be adapted (most patients with IAH and secondary ARDS will have a PAOP above 18 mm Hg).
- IAH increases lung edema; therefore monitoring of extravascular lung water index (EVLWI) seems warranted.[71]
- The combination of capillary leak, positive fluid balance, and raised IAP put the patient at exponential risk for lung edema.
- Body position affects IAP.
  - Putting an obese patient in the upright position can cause ACS.[72]
  - The abdomen should hang freely during prone positioning.[73]
  - The reverse Trendelenburg position may improve respiratory mechanics, however it can decrease splanchnic perfusion.[74]
- Consideration of neuromuscular blockade should balance the potentially beneficial effects on abdominal muscle tone resulting in decreased IAP and improved APP against the potentially detrimental effect on lung mechanics resulting in atelectasis and super-infection.[75]
- The presence of IAH will lead to pulmonary hypertension via increased ITP with direct compression on lung parenchyma and vessels and via the diminished left and right ventricular compliance.
- The effect of IAP on parenchymal compression is exacerbated in cases of hemorrhagic shock or hypotension.

Hepatic Function

The liver appears to be particularly susceptible to injury in the presence of elevated IAP. Animal and human studies have shown impairment of hepatic cell function and liver perfusion even with only moderately elevated IAP of 10 mm Hg.[76,77] Furthermore, acute liver failure, decompensated chronic liver disease, and liver transplantation are frequently complicated by IAH and the ACS.[78,79]

- Close monitoring and early recognition of IAH, followed by aggressive treatment may confer an outcome benefit in patients with liver disease.
- In the management of these patients it might be useful to measure the plasma disappearance rate (PDR) for indocyanine green (ICG), as this correlates not only with liver function and perfusion but also with IAP.[73,80]
- Since cytochrome P450 function may be altered in case of IAH/ACS, medication doses should be adapted accordingly.
- Within the capsule of the liver itself, local hematoma formation may have an adverse affect on tissue perfusion causing a local hepatic compartment syndrome.
- With increasing IAP there is decreased hepatic arterial flow, decreased venous portal flow, and increase in the portacollateral circulation. In turn, physiologic effects include
  - decreased lactate clearance
  - altered glucose metabolism
  - altered mitochondrial function.

Renal Function

IAH has been associated with renal impairment for over 150 years.[81] It is only recently however that a clinically recognized relationship has been found.[82,83] An increasing number of large clinical studies have identified that IAH ($\geq$15 mm Hg) is independently associated with renal impairment and increased mortality.[84,85] The etiology of these changes is not entirely well established; however, it may be multifactorial: reduced renal perfusion, reduced cardiac output, and increased systemic vascular resistance and alterations in humoral and neurogenic factors. Elevated IAP significantly decreases renal venous and arterial blood flow leading to renal dysfunction and failure.[86] Oliguria develops at an IAP of 15 mm Hg and anuria at 30 mm Hg in the presence of normovolemia and at lower levels of IAP in the patient with hypovolemia or sepsis.[87,88] Renal perfusion pressure (RPP) and renal filtration gradient (FG) have been proposed as key factors in the development of IAP-induced renal failure.

- $RPP = MAP - IAP$
- $FG = GFP - PTP = (MAP - IAP) - IAP = MAP - 2 \cdot IAP$
  - Where GFP = glomerular filtration pressure
  - And PTP = proximal tubular pressure

Thus, changes in IAP have a greater impact on renal function and urine production than will changes in MAP. It should not be surprising, therefore, that decreased renal function, as evidenced by development of oliguria, is one of the first visible signs of IAH. Conversely, therefore, it behooves us as clinicians to be cognizant that elevated IAP and its effect on renal function is often the first sign of impending ACS. Other key points to remember are

- The prerenal azotemia seen in IAH is unresponsive to volume expansion to a normal CO, dopaminergic agents, or loop diuretics.[2,89]
- Renal function may be improved by paracentesis of ascitic fluid and reduction in the IAP.[90]
- Prompt reduction of IAP has dramatic beneficial effect on urine output in patients with primary and secondary ACS after trauma.[91–96]

- Within the capsule of the kidney itself, local hematoma formation may have an adverse affect on tissue perfusion causing a local renal compartment syndrome.[97,98]

Gastrointestinal Function

IAH has profound effects on splanchnic organs, causing diminished perfusion, mucosal acidosis, and setting the stage for multiple organ failure.[99] The pathologic changes are more pronounced after sequential insults of ischemia-reperfusion and IAH. It appears that IAH and ACS may serve as the second insult in the two-hit phenomenon of the causation of multiple-organ dysfunction syndrome.[100,101] Recent clinical studies have demonstrated a temporal relationship between ACS and subsequent multiple organ failure (MOF).[99,102,103] In animals, ACS provokes cytokine release and neutrophil migration, resulting in remote organ failure. In humans, ACS results in splanchnic hypoperfusion that may occur in the absence of hypotension or decreased cardiac output. This ischemia and reperfusion injury to the gut serves as a second insult in a two-hit model of MOF where the lymph flow conducts gut-derived proinflammatory cytokines to remote organs.

- IAP inversely correlates with intramucosal (pHi) or regional CO_2.[104–106]
- IAP inversely correlates with indocyanine green plasma disappearance rate (ICG-PDR).[80]
- IAH triggers a vicious cycle leading to intestinal edema, ischemia, bacterial translocation, and finally MOF.[107–109]
- Maintenance of adequate perfusion pressure (APP >60–65 mm Hg) is mandatory.[63]
- The back pressure at the venous side is even more important to the pressure-flow relations.

Abdominal Wall and Endocrine Function

Increased IAP has been shown to reduce abdominal wall blood flow by the direct, compressive effects leading to local ischemia and edema.[110] This can decrease abdominal wall compliance and exacerbate IAH.[69] Abdominal wall muscle and fascial ischemia may contribute to infectious and noninfectious wound complications (eg, dehiscence, herniation, necrotizing fasciitis) often seen in this patient population.

IMPORTANCE OF INTRA-ABDOMINAL PRESSURE IN OTHER CLINICAL CONDITIONS
Abdominal Compartment Syndrome in Pediatric Patients

Omphalocele and gastroschisis are the original clinical conditions that are closely associated with the phenomenon of increased IAP.[111,112] We owe a debt of gratitude to the pediatric surgeons who were the first to deal with defects of the abdominal wall and the consequences of their closure.[113] Several series from the past decade document the manifestations of elevated IAP in children undergoing such repairs, the beneficial effects of monitoring IAP, and the role of elevated IAP in the increased incidence of necrotizing enterocolitis. Please pay attention to IAP in children!

Abdominal Compartment Syndrome in Burn Patients

Patients with large burns (50% or greater or with associated inhalation injury) are at risk of developing IAH.[114] Patients with burns on greater than 70% of total body surface area are at risk of developing ACS, particularly if they have a concurrent inhalation injury. The development of IAH and ACS is related to the volume of crystalloid fluid infused during the burn resuscitation and does not require abdominal injury or operation or even the presence of abdominal wall burn eschar.[114–120]

However, these patients have very large burns, often severe inhalation injuries, and frequently die later in their hospitalization from complications of their burns that are unrelated to their ACS.

- Burn patients are at great risk to develop large-volume resuscitation-related secondary ACS.
- Burn patients who develop IAH mostly have more then 50% total body surface area (TBSA) burns.
- A variety of management options exist for IAH and ACS in burn patients, all of which may be of some benefit.[117,120]
  - sedation
  - pharmacologic paralysis
  - abdominal wall escharotomy
  - percutaneous catheter decompression of the peritoneal cavity
  - surgical decompression.

Abdominal Compartment Syndrome in Hematological Patients

Recent studies have alluded to the increased incidence and consequences of IAH in hematological patients,[121] the causes of which are multifactorial:

- Growth factor–induced capillary leak syndrome with concomitant large-volume fluid resuscitation and third-space sequestration
- Chemotherapy-induced ileus, colonic pseudo-obstruction (Ogilvie's syndrome), mucositis, or gastroenteritis
- Sepsis and infectious complications aggravating intestinal and capillary permeability
- Extramedullary hematopoiesis as seen with chronic myeloid leukemia resulting in hepatosplenomegaly, chronic IAH, and chronic (irreversible) pulmonary hypertension
- The mechanisms of veno-occlusive disease seen after stem cell transplantation may be triggered by or related to increased IAP.

Abdominal Compartment Syndrome in Morbidly Obese Patients

Recent studies show that obese patients have higher baseline IAP values.[122] As with IAH in the critically ill, elevated IAP in the morbidly obese patient can have far-reaching effects on end-organ function. Disease processes common in morbidly obese patients such as obesity hypoventilation syndrome, pseudotumor cerebri, gastroesophageal reflux, and stress urinary incontinence are now being recognized as being caused by the increased IAP occurring with an elevated body mass index.[13,42,123] Furthermore, the increased incidence of poor fascial healing and incisional hernia rates have been related to the IAH-induced reductions in rectus sheath and abdominal wall blood flow.

- IAH-related complications of morbid obesity generally respond to weight loss.[44]
- The morbidly obese are at a greater risk of developing ACS because of preexisting baseline IAH and organ dysfunction.
- Clinicians should have a low threshold for monitoring IAP in obese patients because of the so-called "silent IAH."

Intra-Abdominal Pressure During Pregnancy

In the second and the third trimesters of pregnancy, the uterus occupies a major part of the abdominal cavity, and in the supine position breathlessness and blood pressure drop ("supine hypotension syndrome") are seen.[124] These symptoms are the result of restriction of the diaphragm and compression of the inferior vena cava. However, overall IAP is usually not elevated.[125] Furthermore, the symptoms are alleviated in the lateral, sitting, or standing positions. Because of hormonal influences during pregnancy, the abdominal wall is slowly stretched, increasing its compliance, which reduces the potential for increase in IAP caused by the expanding uterus. However, if IAP increases as a result of other reasons, eg, pneumoperitoneum at laparoscopy, perfusion of the uterus and the fetus might be severely compromised.[126]

INTRODUCING A NEW CONCEPT: THE POLYCOMPARTMENT SYNDROME

Within a specific compartment, the CS can be localized like a pelvic compartment syndrome or global like ACS; thus, we suggest the terms localized CS (LCS) and global CS (GCS). Scalea and colleagues[127] alluded to the term multiple compartment syndrome (MCS) in a study of 102 patients with increased intra-abdominal (IAP), intrathoracic, and intracranial pressure (ICP) after severe brain injury. Seventy-eight patients had an ICS and underwent a decompressive craniectomy (DC). The DC in these 78 patients resulted in a significant decrease in ICP from 24 to 14 mm Hg. The other 24 patients had a multiple CS and underwent both a decompressive craniectomy and a decompressive laparotomy (DL). The combination of DC and DL in these 24 patients led to a decrease in ICP from around 32 to 14 mm Hg after DC and from 28 to 19 mm Hg after DL (the effect being different depending on whether DC or DL was performed first). After DL, the IAP decreased from 28 to around 18 mm Hg and so did mean airway pressure from 37 to 27 cmH2O. The authors concluded that increased ICP can result from primary traumatic brain injury as well as from increased IAP, which has been documented before.[32,33,128] Patients with multiple CS showed a trend toward higher mortality (42% versus 31%), although it did not reach statistical significance. Multiple CS should therefore be considered in multiple injured patients with increased ICP that does not respond to therapy.[127]

Since the term multi or multiple CS is mostly used in the literature referring to multiple limb trauma with CS needing decompressive fasciotomy and to avoid confusion, the term polycompartment syndrome was finally coined.[129] Because of the central position of the abdomen and the effects of IAP on nearly all other compartments, IAH and ACS play a central role in the development of poly CS (**Fig. 3**). The increased IAP hence will affect ICP, ITP, CVP, and PAOP.

FLUID RESUSCITATION, MULTIPLE ORGAN FAILURE, AND POLYCOMPARTMENT SYNDROME

Clearly the relationship between fluid resuscitation and IAH is very complex since fluid overload is a leading cause of IAH, but fluid loading may also protect against some of the detrimental effects of IAH on organ function. Therefore, we dedicate a section of this article to this complex issue.

Why Do We Like Fluids?

The importance of increasing circulating blood volume in hypovolemic shock has been apparent for decades and the implementation of guidelines and protocols for fluid management in trauma has saved countless lives. After the success obtained in hypovolemic shock, aggressive fluid resuscitation has been studied in distributive shock as well. Burn resuscitation is a well-known example, where mortality was significantly decreased using aggressive crystalloid resuscitation. In septic shock as well, fluid resuscitation is the first and foremost therapeutic action recommended in

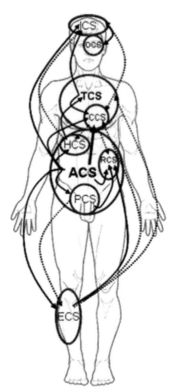

Fig. 3. Interactions between different compartments. The arrows indicate possible interactions between different compartments. Solid lines show direct effects by mechanical pressure forces. Dotted lines show indirect distant effects between compartments. ACS, abdominal compartment syndrome; CCS, cardiac compartment syndrome; ECS, extremity compartment syndrome; HCS, hepatic compartment syndrome; ICS, intracranial compartment syndrome; RCS, renal compartment syndrome; OCS, orbital compartment syndrome; PCS, pelvic compartment syndrome; TCS, thoracic compartment syndrome.

the Surviving Sepsis Campaign Guidelines.[51] Traditionally, fluid resuscitation protocols are aimed at correction of "basic" physiologic parameters such as blood pressure, central venous pressure (CVP), and urine output. The advantages of this approach are multiple and easy to understand: these parameters are readily available at the bedside and do not require expensive and operator-dependent equipment, leading to broader applicability worldwide. Over time, the only significant evolution regarding the use of fluid resuscitation as such has been the gradual increase in emphasis on the importance of time. Both in trauma and burns, delayed fluid resuscitation has been associated with increased mortality. ATLS guidelines as well as burn resuscitation guidelines have stressed the importance of prompt administration of fluids for a long time.[130] The importance of time in sepsis was highlighted more recently in the landmark paper by Rivers and colleagues[52] and current sepsis guidelines have embraced this concept completely.[51]

Which Fluids Do We Like?

The goal of fluid resuscitation is to restore circulating blood volume, which may mean substitution of external losses, supplying volume to a dilated vascular system, or

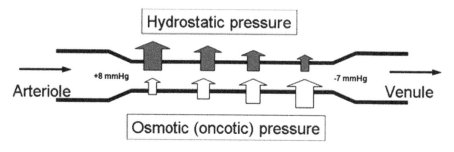

Force	Pressure	Arteriole	Venule
INTO interstitium	P_c	30 mmHg	15 mmHg
	π_i	6 mmHg	6 mmHg
INTO capillaries	π_c	- 28 mmHg	- 28 mmHg
	P_i	- 0 mmHg	- 0 mmHg
	Net pressure	+ 8 mmHg	-7 mmHg
		INTO interstitium	INTO capillaries

$$J_v = K_f([P_c - P_i] - \sigma[\pi_c - \pi_i])$$

Fig. 4. The Starling equation. Capillaries act rather like a leaky hosepipe: although the bulk of the fluid continues along the pipe, the pressure forces come out of the walls. Hydrostatic (blood) pressure is not the only force acting to cause fluid movement in and out of the capillaries. The plasma proteins that cannot cross the capillary walls exert an osmotic pressure to draw water back into the capillaries, which outweighs the hydrostatic pressure at the venous end of the capillaries. The net pressure at the arteriolar site is +8 mm Hg and forces fluids into the interstitium; the net pressure at the venular site is −7 mm Hg and drives fluids back into the capillaries. Each day about 20 L is lost while 16 L is regained. J_v is the net fluid movement between compartments The other factors are: Capillary hydrostatic pressure (P_c) Interstitial hydrostatic pressure (P_i) Capillary oncotic pressure (π_c) Interstitial oncotic pressure (π_i) Filtration coefficient (K_f) Reflection coefficient (σ).

supplementing internal losses due to third spacing or capillary leak. This has traditionally been accomplished using isotonic crystalloid solutions, which contain mainly NaCl. Since the Na+ ion is an extracellular ion, crystalloid solutions will be evenly distributed throughout the extracellular body water compartment after intravenous (IV) administration. In the search for fluids that would selectively expand the intravascular compartment, colloids, both synthetic and natural, were evaluated. According to Starling's equation, they should tip the balance in favor of fluid movement from the interstitial to the intravascular compartment and thus plasma volume expansion (**Fig. 4**). However, several studies could not show a survival benefit in favor of colloid resuscitation using either albumin or synthetic colloid solutions in several clinical situations. Furthermore, colloids are more expensive; albumin and gelatins were manufactured as derivatives from human and animal tissue and therefore carried a small risk for disease transmission; and synthetic colloids were associated with adverse effects such as anaphylaxis, renal failure, and coagulation defects. These findings resulted in the incorporation of crystalloid solutions in guidelines as the gold standard for fluid resuscitation, especially in North American literature and guidelines. This has led to administration of enormous amounts of crystalloid solution in the first 24 hours after major trauma, burns, or septic shock. In several studies, mean administration of more than 30 L of crystalloids over 24 hours has been reported! In situations associated with capillary leak, this approach leads to development of massive tissue edema and the iatrogenic complications that ensue may lead to the polycompartment syndrome and multiple organ failure and death. Reports of mortality secondary to massive fluid resuscitation after trauma or shock are appearing increasingly over the past 10 years.

Do We Like Fluids Too Much?

The dangers of underresuscitation in terms of amount or timing of fluid administration are clear, but the adverse effects of overresuscitation, especially using crystalloids, are only recently being recognized. There is increasing evidence that increased compartment pressures and especially IAH may be the missing link between overresuscitation, multiple organ failure, and death.[131] As early as 1999, IAH and ACS were described in patients who received massive fluid resuscitation after extra-abdominal injury.[132] The mechanism through which massive fluid resuscitation causes IAH is probably related to capillary leak and edema, both of the abdominal wall (leading to decreased abdominal wall compliance) and of the bowel wall (leading to increased abdominal volume). In a retrospective series by Maxwell and colleagues,[132] the incidence of abdominal decompression among non–abdominal trauma victims was found to be 0.5%. The mean amount of fluids administered was 19 $\pm$ 5 L of crystalloid and 29 $\pm$ 10 units of packed red blood cells, the mortality was 67%, and nonsurvivors were decompressed approximately 20 hours later than survivors. The authors suggested that the incidence of secondary ACS may be higher than previously thought in non–abdominal trauma victims and that early decompression may improve outcome since some improvement in organ function after decompression was seen. They recommended IAP monitoring in patients receiving high amounts of fluid resuscitation. A landmark paper by Balogh and colleagues[133] confirmed these findings. In their series, 11 (9%) of 128 standardized shock resuscitation patients developed secondary ACS. All cases were recognized and decompressed within 24 hours of hospital admission. After decompression, the bladder pressure and the systemic vascular resistance decreased, while the mean arterial pressure, cardiac index, and static lung compliance increased. The mortality rate was 54%. Those who died failed to respond to decompression with increased cardiac index and a sustained decrease in IAP. In analogy to trauma, secondary ACS has since been described also in burns and sepsis. The multiple-center studies on the prevalence and incidence of IAH in mixed ICU patients also showed that a positive net fluid balance as well as a positive cumulative fluid balance were predictors for poor outcome: nonsurvivors had a positive cumulative fluid balance of about 6 L versus 1 L in survivors.[25,26] Similar results have also been found by Alsous and colleagues:[134] at least 1 day of negative fluid balance (≤ -500 mL) achieved by the third day of treatment was a good independent predictor of survival in patients with septic shock. Very recently, Daugherty and colleagues[135] conducted a prospective cohort study among 468 medical ICU patients. Forty patients (8.5%) had a net positive fluid balance of more than 5 L after 24 hours (after all risk factors for primary ACS served as exclusion criteria). The incidence of IAH in this group was a staggering 85% and 25% developed secondary ACS. The study was not powered to detect differences in mortality and outcome parameters were not statistically different between patients with or without IAH and ACS. Nevertheless, there was a trend toward higher mortality in the IAH groups and mortality figures reached 80% in the ACS group. Although epidemiologic research regarding this subject is virtually nonexistent, the increase in reported series seems to indicate increasing incidence of this highly lethal complication. In light of this increasing body of evidence regarding the association between massive fluid resuscitation, intra-abdominal hypertension, organ dysfunction, and mortality, it seems wise to at least incorporate IAP as a parameter in all future studies regarding fluid management, and to put into question current clinical practice guidelines, not in terms of whether to administer fluids at all, but in terms of the parameters we use to guide our treatment.

So How Should We Use Our Fluids?

As a result of the increasing problems with massive fluid resuscitation, many researchers have gone back to the concept of small volume resuscitation. This concept, to achieve the same physiologic goals as in "classical" crystalloid resuscitation using smaller volumes, implies the use of hypertonic or hyperosmotic solutions. In the American literature there is growing interest in the use of hypertonic saline for several indications.[136,137] The European literature and clinical practice, having never abandoned colloid administration completely, has focused mainly on new synthetic colloids such as 130-kD hydroxyethyl starch (HES – Voluven). Attempts to combine both strategies have led to several studies using mixed hypertonic saline and colloid infusions, eg, hyperHES, a solution consisting of NaCl 7.2% in HES with mixed results. Although good results have been obtained with small-volume resuscitation in most of these studies, many of them unfortunately make no mention of IAP or incidence of IAH and ACS at all. In the area of burn resuscitation there are some exceptions: Oda and colleagues[138] did report a reduced risk for abdominal compartment syndrome (as well as lower fluid requirements during the first 24 hours and lower peak inspiratory pressures after 24 hours) when using hypertonic lactated saline for burn resuscitation and O'Mara and colleagues[139] reported lower fluid requirements and lower IAP using colloids.

INTRODUCING ANOTHER NEW CONCEPT: ACUTE BOWEL INJURY AND ACUTE INTESTINAL DISTRESS SYNDROME

Although few epidemiologic data are available to confirm this observation, it is our impression that the incidence of primary IAH/ACS is decreasing owing to increased awareness of the problem among surgeons, who are more likely to leave the abdomen open in high-risk surgery cases.[140–142] This observation was also mentioned by Kimball and colleagues[143] in a series of ruptured aortic aneurysm cases and in a recent survey.[144]

The focus of attention is shifting to secondary ACS and rightfully so. This syndrome is highly prevalent in critically ill patients and leads to even higher mortality than primary IAH. As described by Kimball and colleagues[143] and Kirkpatrick and colleagues,[145] a variety of noxious stimuli (such as infection, trauma, burns, and sepsis) can lead to activation of the innate immune system and neutrophil activation. This systemic immune response causes release of cytokines into the circulation leading to systemic inflammatory response syndrome (SIRS) and capillary leak. Apart from direct negative impact on cellular organ function, this syndrome also exerts its deleterious effect through accumulation of extravascular fluids in the tissues and local ischemia. This mechanism of injury is widely recognized and accepted in the lung, where it is classified as acute lung injury (ALI) or acute respiratory distress syndrome (ARDS). However, the same pathologic process occurs in the gut, but this concept is much slower to seep into general ICU practice.

Why is this the case? It is undoubtedly true that bowel function is much harder to quantify than, for example, lung function. PaO2/FiO2 ratios are very easy to calculate at the bedside and monitoring parameters such as extravascular lung water index (EVLWI) have been demonstrated to be accurate prognostic predictors. However, the role of the gut as the motor of organ dysfunction syndrome cannot be denied and difficulties in assessing gut function should not deter us from recognizing that

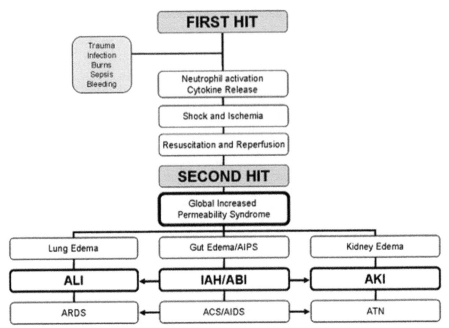

Fig. 5. The two-hit model causing the polycompartment syndrome. ABI, acute bowel injury; ACS, abdominal compartment syndrome; AIDS, acute intestinal distress syndrome; AIPS, acute intestinal permeability syndrome; AKI, acute kidney injury; ALI, acute lung injury; ARDS, acute respiratory distress syndrome; ATN, acute tubular necrosis; IAH, intra-abdominal hypertension.

concept. In fact, in analogy to ALI and AKI, we propose the introduction of a concept named acute bowel injury (ABI), which is manifested through bowel edema and the ensuing IAH. Even more than other organ dysfunction syndromes, ABI goes hand in hand with the polycompartment syndrome and has a negative impact on distant organ systems through the development of IAH, and can contribute to the development of AKI and ALI.

HOW DO WE DEFINE ACUTE BOWEL INJURY AND ACUTE INTESTINAL DISTRESS SYNDROME?

No specific markers of bowel function have been identified, apart from the very crude on/off parameter of enteral feeding tolerance. However, since capillary leak and bowel edema are cornerstones of this syndrome, ABI can probably best been defined in terms of IAP levels. Another plus for IAP is that it has already been linked to prognosis in several epidemiologic studies. One might argue than that the ABI concept is just another word for IAH. However, ABI reflects a more basic concept of complex bowel injury caused by a first hit (either directly, such as in abdominal sepsis or trauma, or indirectly such as in ischemia due to hypovolemic or distributive shock), followed by a second hit in the form of capillary leak, bowel edema, and local ischemia, of which (secondary) IAH is the result (**Fig. 5**). If the vicious cycle is not stopped this will eventually lead to acute intestinal distress syndrome (AIDS) and ACS. In the light of the increased permeability as the motor of the first and second hit some suggested the term acute intestinal permeability syndrome (AIPS). This can evolve to a more

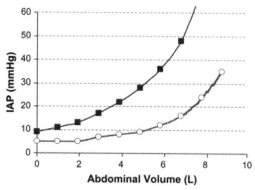

Fig. 6. Pressure volume curves of the abdomen in a patient with poor abdominal wall compliance (*closed squares*) compared with a patient with normal (*open circles*) abdominal wall compliance. (*Adapted from* Malbrain ML. Different techniques to measure intra-abdominal pressure (IAP): time for a critical re-appraisal. Intensive Care Med 2004;30:357–71; with permission.)

intuitive understanding of the complexity of the pathologic process instead of a purely mechanical viewpoint of increased pressure in a confined anatomic space.

CLINICAL MANAGEMENT

The management of patients with IAH is based on the following four principles:[27,146,147]

- specific procedures to reduce IAP and the consequences of ACS
- general support (intensive care) of the critically ill patient
- surgical decompression
- optimization after surgical decompression to perhaps counteract some of the specific adverse effects associated with decompression.

Medical Treatment

Before surgical decompression is considered, less invasive medical treatment options should be optimized. The relation between abdominal contents and IAP is not linear but exponential (**Fig. 6**) and this curve is shifted to the left and upward when abdominal wall compliance is decreased. Therefore IAH can be treated by improving abdominal wall compliance and by decreasing intra-abdominal volume or both. Different medical treatments have been suggested to decrease IAP.[64] These are based on five different mechanisms:

- Improvement of abdominal wall compliance
- Evacuation of intraluminal contents
- Evacuation of abdominal fluid collections
- Correction of capillary leak and positive fluid balance
- Specific treatments.

An algorithm for the clinical management of IAH and ACS is proposed in **Fig. 7**. **Box 2** gives an overview of the different medical treatment options.

Improvement of abdominal wall compliance

Sedation can help to control IAH by increasing abdominal wall compliance. Neuromuscular blockade has also been shown to decrease IAP, a phenomenon known for

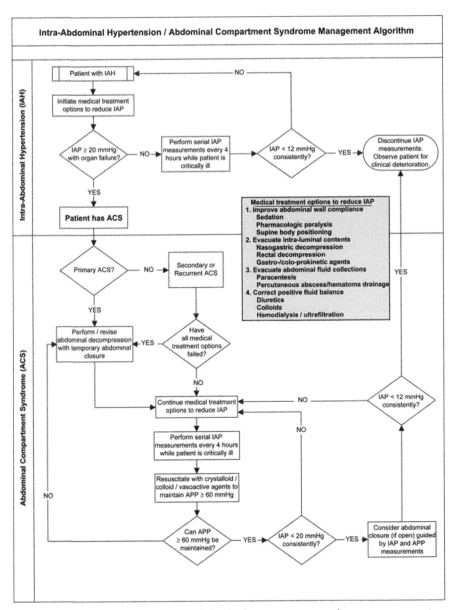

Fig. 7. Intra-abdominal hypertension/abdominal compartment syndrome management.

a long time in the operating theater.[33,75,148–150] Fentanyl, on the contrary, may acutely increase IAP by stimulation of active phasic expiratory activity.[151] Body positioning and the use of skin pressure decreasing interfaces will also affect IAP.[73,74,80] A percutaneous procedure to increase abdominal capacity/compliance and to decrease IAP, based on the principles of abdominal wall components separation was recently validated in a porcine ACS model.[152] In burn patients, a similar procedure had the same beneficial effects.[120]

Box 2
Medical treatment options for IAH and ACS

Improvement of abdominal wall compliance

- Sedation
- Pain relief (not fentanyl!)
- Neuromuscular blockade
- Body positioning
- Negative fluid balance
- Skin pressure decreasing interfaces
- Weight loss
- Percutaneous abdominal wall component separation

Evacuation of intraluminal contents

- Gastric tube and suctioning
- Gastroprokinetics (erythromycin, cisapride, metoclopramide)
- Rectal tube and enemas
- Colonoprokinetics (neostygmine, prostygmine bolus, or infusion)
- Endoscopic decompression of large bowel
- Colostomy
- Ileostomy

Evacuation of peri-intestinal and abdominal fluids

- Ascites evacuation
- CT- or ultrasound (US)-guided aspiration of abscess
- CT- or US-guided aspiration of hematoma
- Percutaneous drainage of (blood) collections

Correction of capillary leak and positive fluid balance

- Albumin in combination with diuretics (furosemide)
- Correction of capillary leak (eg, antibiotics, source control)
- Colloids instead of crystalloids
- Dobutamine (not dopamine!)
- Dialysis or CVVH with ultrafiltration
- Ascorbinic acid in burn patients

Specific therapeutic interventions

- Continuous negative abdominal pressure (CNAP)
- Negative external abdominal pressure (NEXAP)
- Targeted abdominal perfusion pressure (APP)
- (experimental: Octreotide and melatonin in ACS)

Evacuation of intra-luminal contents

Ileus is common in most critically ill patients. Noninvasive evacuation of abdominal contents should be tried by means of gastric tube placement and suctioning, rectal tube, and enemas and possibly endoscopic decompression.[153–156] This can be done in conjunction with gastro- and or colonoprokinetics such as erythromycin (200 mg IV every 6 hours), metoclopramide (10 mg IV every 8 hours), neostygmine or prostygmine (2 mg diluted in up to 50 mL iv given slowly by infusion).[157–162]

Evacuation of abdominal fluid collections

Drainage of tense ascites may result in a decrease in IAP.[90,163–166] In patients with liver cirrhosis and esophageal varices, paracentesis helps to decrease variceal wall tension and the risk for rupture and bleeding.[167] Paracentesis is also the treatment of choice in burn patients with secondary ACS.[120,168,169] In the case of hematomas, blood collections, or a local abscess, CT-guided fine-needle aspiration has recently been described in the setting of IAH and ACS.

Correction of capillary leak and positive fluid balance

In the initial phase of ACS, fluid loss should be compensated to prevent splanchnic hypoperfusion.[58,170,171] Low-dose infusion of dobutamine, but not dopamine, also corrects the intestinal mucosal perfusion impairment induced by moderate increases in intra-abdominal pressure.[172] Because of the nature of the illness and injury associated with ACS, these patients retain large volumes of sodium and water. Because of the capillary leak this will exacerbate tissue edema and third spacing, creating a vicious cycle of ongoing IAH. In the early stages, diuretic therapy in combination with albumin can be considered to mobilize the edema, but only if the patient is hemodynamically stable. Many patients, however, will develop anuria as renal blood flow is reduced. In these cases, the institution of renal replacement therapy should not be delayed, with fluid removal by intermittent dialysis or CVVH.[173–175]

Specific treatments

Recently the application of continuous negative abdominal pressure by means of a cuirass has been studied in animals and humans showing a decrease in IAP and increase in end-expiratory lung volumes.[34,38,176–178]

In a similar manner to targeting cerebral perfusion pressure (CPP = MAP − ICP) or coronary perfusion pressure (CoPP = DBP − PAOP), it may be appropriate to target abdominal perfusion pressure (APP), where APP = MAP − IAP, to a level that reduces the risk of worsened splanchnic perfusion and subsequent organ dysfunction.[48,63,64]

Octreotide, a long-acting somatostatin analog, has been studied primarily in animals and has shown ability to control neutrophil infiltration and improve the reperfusion-induced oxidative damage after decompression of secondary intra-abdominal hypertension.[179]

Melatonin, a secretory product of the pineal gland known to have free radical scavenging and antioxidative properties, has recently shown ability to reduce lipid peroxidation in cell membranes, a process that promotes cell death, as the functional integrity of these structures is damage.[180]

Surgical Decompression

Although decompression remains the only definite management for ACS, the timing of this procedure still remains controversial. During the intervention, specific anesthetic challenges need to be solved and after decompression the patient is at risk for ischemia reperfusion injury, venous stasis, and fatal pulmonary embolism.[181] Maintaining adequate preload and abdominal perfusion pressure are the keys to success.[49,58,63] Open abdomen treatment (or laparostomy) was initially intended for patients with diffuse intra-abdominal infections, and often used in combination with a planned relaparotomy approach. Because of the increased awareness of the deleterious effects of intra-abdominal hypertension, open abdomen treatment, either prophylactic or therapeutic, is more common nowadays in the ICU.[102,182]

Several methods for temporary abdominal closure (TAC) are available, but their detailed description lies beyond the scope of this text.[183] Although open abdomen treatment can be complicated by delayed fascial closure, enterocutaneous fistulae, wound infections, and intractable fluid losses, leading to frequent reoperations and longer ICU stay, a large study has shown that the decreased mental, physical, emotional, and behavioral health status after decompressive laparotomy returns to that of the general population after 1 year.[184]

SUMMARY

First suggested in 1863 by Marey, ACS is the end stage of the physiologic sequellae of increased IAP, termed IAH. Recent observations suggest an increasing frequency of this complication in all types of patients. Even chronic elevations of IAP seem to affect the various organ systems in the body. The presence of IAH and ACS are significant causes of organ failure, increased resource use, decreased economic productivity, and increased mortality among a wide variety of patient populations.[25,29] Despite its obvious clinical implications, too little attention is paid to IAP, IAH, and ACS. Although there is much research interest in the subject, there are still too many unanswered questions that cloud our understanding of the pathophysiology of this syndrome.

In analogy to AKI and ALI, there is certainly a need for basic research into the underlying mechanisms of the new concepts of acute bowel injury and the polycompartment syndrome. Ischemia/reperfusion injury research in particular seems to show a lot of promise into this pathogenesis. At the same time, clinical research is also necessary.

Currently no good multicentric randomized interventional controlled clinical trial has tackled the question of whether an increase of IAP is a phenomenon or an epiphenomenon and whether any intervention to normalize IAP or APP will eventually affect patient outcome. Until that study exists, there will always be believers and nonbelievers.[185] The development of a management algorithm for IAH/ACS compares with the multifaceted approach emerging for early goal-directed therapy in sepsis.[52] The world society of the abdominal compartment syndrome (WSACS) invites interested researchers to join the society, to adhere to the consensus definitions posted at the Web site, and to submit some prospective data for the next world congress (www.wcacs.org), to be held in Dublin, Ireland, June 24 to 27, 2009. For those who carry the mandate to future IAH/ACS research, the path ahead is clear: using available evidence, we must develop an IAH/ACS therapeutic bundle and apply it in a multiple center, prospective, outcome trial. In a separate effort, attempts should be made to better understand the causes and evolution of ABI, AIDS/AIPS, and the polycompartment syndrome. In our opinion, it is one of the great scientific adventures of the future to link all the data that we have today on organ dysfunction, be it ALI, AKI, or ABI, and bring them together in a single broad-based concept that can explain the different aspects of the systemic inflammatory response syndrome and provide clues for treatment, not only aimed at the organs involved, but at the core of what kills our patients.

REFERENCES

1. Malbrain ML, Cheatham ML, Kirkpatrick A, et al. Results from the International Conference of experts on intra-abdominal hypertension and abdominal compartment syndrome. I. Definitions. Intensive Care Med 2006;32:1722–32.
2. Fietsam R Jr, Villalba M, Glover JL, et al. Intra-abdominal compartment syndrome as a complication of ruptured abdominal aortic aneurysm repair. Am Surg 1989;55:396–402.
3. Malbrain ML, De laet I, Cheatham M. Consensus conference definitions and recommendations on intra-abdominal hypertension (IAH) and the abdominal compartment syndrome (ACS)—the long road to the final publications, how did we get there? Acta Clin Belg Suppl 2007;62:44–59.

4. Malbrain ML, Cheatham ML, Kirkpatrick A, et al. Abdominal compartment syndrome: it's time to pay attention! Intensive Care Med 2006;32:1912–4.

5. Malbrain ML. You don't have any excuse, just start measuring abdominal pressure and act upon it! Minerva Anestesiol 2008;74:1–2.

6. Ivatury RR. Abdominal compartment syndrome: a century later, isn't it time to accept and promulgate? Crit Care Med 2006;34:2494–5.

7. Kirkpatrick AW, Brenneman FD, McLean RF, et al. Is clinical examination an accurate indicator of raised intra-abdominal pressure in critically injured patients? Can J Surg 2000;43:207–11.

8. Sugrue M, Bauman A, Jones F, et al. Clinical examination is an inaccurate predictor of intraabdominal pressure. World J Surg 2002;26:1428–31.

9. Malbrain ML. Different techniques to measure intra-abdominal pressure (IAP): time for a critical re-appraisal. Intensive Care Med 2004;30:357–71.

10. Malbrain M, Jones F. Intra-abdominal pressure measurement techniques. In: Ivatury R, Cheatham M, Malbrain M, et al. Abdominal compartment syndrome. Georgetown (TX): Landes Bioscience; 2006. p. 19–68.

11. Sanchez NC, Tenofsky PL, Dort JM, et al. What is normal intra-abdominal pressure? Am Surg 2001;67:243–8.

12. Sugerman H, Windsor A, Bessos M, et al. Intra-abdominal pressure, sagittal abdominal diameter and obesity comorbidity. J Intern Med 1997;241:71–9.

13. Sugerman HJ. Effects of increased intra-abdominal pressure in severe obesity. 2001;81:1063–75, vi.

14. Davis PJ, Koottayi S, Taylor A, et al. Comparison of indirect methods of measuring intra-abdominal pressure in children. Intensive Care Med 2005;31:471–5.

15. Saggi B, Ivatury R, Sugerman HJ. Surgical critical care issues: abdominal compartment syndrome. In: Holzheimer RG, Mannick JA, editors. Surgical treatment evidence-based and problem-oriented. München: W. Zuckschwerdt Verlag München; 2001.

16. De Potter TJ, Dits H, Malbrain ML. Intra- and interobserver variability during in vitro validation of two novel methods for intra-abdominal pressure monitoring. Intensive Care Med 2005;31:747–51.

17. De Waele J, Pletinckx P, Blot S, et al. Saline volume in transvesical intra-abdominal pressure measurement: enough is enough. Intensive Care Med 2006;32:455–9.

18. Malbrain ML, Deeren DH. Effect of bladder volume on measured intravesical pressure: a prospective cohort study. Crit Care 2006;10:R98.

19. Ball CG, Kirkpatrick AW. 'Progression towards the minimum': the importance of standardizing the priming volume during the indirect measurement of intra-abdominal pressures. Crit Care 2006;10:153.

20. De laet I, Hoste E, De Waele JJ. Transvesical intra-abdominal pressure measurement using minimal instillation volumes: how low can we go? Intensive Care Med 2008;34:746–50.

21. Malbrain ML. The assumed problem of air bubbles in the tubing during intra-abdominal pressure measurement—author reply. Intensive Care Med 2004;30:1693.

22. Schachtrupp A, Henzler D, Orfao S, et al. Evaluation of a modified piezoresistive technique and a water-capsule technique for direct and continuous measurement of intra-abdominal pressure in a porcine model. Crit Care Med 2006;34:745–50.

23. Schachtrupp A, Tons C, Fackeldey V, et al. Evaluation of two novel methods for the direct and continuous measurement of the intra-abdominal pressure in a porcine model. Intensive Care Med 2003;29:1605–8.

24. Balogh Z, Jones F, D'Amours S, et al. Continuous intra-abdominal pressure measurement technique. Am J Surg 2004;188:679–84.
25. Malbrain ML, Chiumello D, Pelosi P, et al. Incidence and prognosis of intraabdominal hypertension in a mixed population of critically ill patients: a multiple-center epidemiological study. Crit Care Med 2005;33:315–22.
26. Malbrain ML, Chiumello D, Pelosi P, et al. Prevalence of intra-abdominal hypertension in critically ill patients: a multicentre epidemiological study. Intensive Care Med 2004;30:822–9.
27. Cheatham ML, Malbrain ML, Kirkpatrick A, et al. Results from the International Conference of experts on intra-abdominal hypertension and abdominal compartment syndrome. II. Recommendations. Intensive Care Med 2007;33:951–62.
28. Suominen PK, Pakarinen MP, Rautiainen P, et al. Comparison of direct and intra-vesical measurement of intraabdominal pressure in children. J Pediatr Surg 2006;41:1381–5.
29. Malbrain ML. Is it wise not to think about intraabdominal hypertension in the ICU? Curr Opin Crit Care 2004;10:132–45.
30. Malbrain ML, Deeren D, De Potter TJ. Intra-abdominal hypertension in the critically ill: it is time to pay attention. Curr Opin Crit Care 2005;11:156–71.
31. Citerio G, Berra L. Central nervous system. In: Ivatury R, Cheatham M, Malbrain M, et al, editors. Abdominal compartment syndrome. Georgetown (TX): Landes Bioscience; 2006. p. 144–56.
32. Citerio G, Vascotto E, Villa F, et al. Induced abdominal compartment syndrome increases intracranial pressure in neurotrauma patients: a prospective study. Crit Care Med 2001;29:1466–71.
33. Deeren D, Dits H, Malbrain MLNG. Correlation between intra-abdominal and intra-cranial pressure in nontraumatic brain injury. Intensive Care Med 2005;31:1577–81.
34. Bloomfield G, Saggi B, Blocher C, et al. Physiologic effects of externally applied continuous negative abdominal pressure for intra-abdominal hypertension. 1999;46:1009–14 [discussion: 14–6].
35. Bloomfield GL, Dalton JM, Sugerman HJ, et al. Treatment of increasing intracranial pressure secondary to the acute abdominal compartment syndrome in a patient with combined abdominal and head trauma. J Trauma 1995;39:1168–70.
36. Bloomfield GL, Ridings PC, Blocher CR, et al. Effects of increased intra-abdominal pressure upon intracranial and cerebral perfusion pressure before and after volume expansion. J Trauma 1996;40:936–41 [discussion: 41–3].
37. Bloomfield GL, Ridings PC, Blocher CR, et al. A proposed relationship between increased intra-abdominal, intrathoracic, and intracranial pressure. Crit Care Med 1997;25:496–503.
38. Saggi BH, Bloomfield GL, Sugerman HJ, et al. Treatment of intracranial hypertension using nonsurgical abdominal decompression. J Trauma 1999;46:646–51.
39. Irgau I, Koyfman Y, Tikellis JI. Elective intraoperative intracranial pressure monitoring during laparoscopic cholecystectomy. Arch Surg 1995;130:1011–3.
40. Joseph DK, Dutton RP, Aarabi B, et al. Decompressive laparotomy to treat intractable intracranial hypertension after traumatic brain injury. J Trauma 2004;57:687–93 [discussion: 93–5].
41. Josephs LG, Este-McDonald JR, Birkett DH, et al. Diagnostic laparoscopy increases intracranial pressure. 1994;36:815–8 [discussion: 8–9].
42. Sugerman HJ, DeMaria EJ, Felton WL III, et al. Increased intra-abdominal pressure and cardiac filling pressures in obesity-associated pseudotumor cerebri. Neurology 1997;49:507–11.

43. Sugerman HJ, Felton IW III, Sismanis A, et al. Continuous negative abdominal pressure device to treat pseudotumor cerebri. Int J Obes Relat Metab Disord 2001;25:486–90.

44. Sugerman H, Windsor A, Bessos M, et al. Effects of surgically induced weight loss on urinary bladder pressure, sagittal abdominal diameter and obesity co-morbidity. Int J Obes Relat Metab Disord 1998;22:230–5.

45. Kashtan J, Green JF, Parsons EQ, et al. Hemodynamic effect of increased abdominal pressure. J Surg Res 1981;30:249–55.

46. Ridings PC, Bloomfield GL, Blocher CR, et al. Cardiopulmonary effects of raised intra-abdominal pressure before and after intravascular volume expansion. J Trauma 1995;39:1071–5.

47. Richardson JD, Trinkle JK. Hemodynamic and respiratory alterations with increased intra-abdominal pressure. J Surg Res 1976;20:401–4.

48. Malbrain ML, Cheatham ML. Cardiovascular effects and optimal preload markers in intra-abdominal hypertension. In: Vincent J-L, editor. Yearbook of intensive care and emergency medicine. Berlin: Springer-Verlag; 2004. p. 519–43.

49. Cheatham M, Malbrain M. Abdominal perfusion pressure. In: Ivatury R, Cheatham M, Malbrain M, et al, editors. Abdominal compartment syndrome. Georgetown (TX): Landes Bioscience; 2006;69–81.

50. Cheatham M, Malbrain M. Cardiovascular implications of elevated intra-abdominal pressure. In: Ivatury R, Cheatham M, Malbrain M, et al, editors. Abdominal compartment syndrome. Georgetown (TX): Landes Bioscience; 2006. p. 89–104.

51. Dellinger RP, Carlet JM, Masur H, et al. Surviving Sepsis Campaign guidelines for management of severe sepsis and septic shock. Intensive Care Med 2004;30: 536–55.

52. Rivers E, Nguyen B, Havstad S, et al. Early goal-directed therapy in the treatment of severe sepsis and septic shock. N Engl J Med 2001;345:1368–77.

53. Cheatham ML, Block EF, Nelson LD, et al. Superior predictor of the hemodynamic response to fluid challenge in critically ill patients. Chest 1998;114:1226–7.

54. Cheatham ML, Nelson LD, Chang MC, et al. Right ventricular end-diastolic volume index as a predictor of preload status in patients on positive end-expiratory pressure. Crit Care Med 1998;26:1801–6.

55. Schachtrupp A, Graf J, Tons C, et al. Intravascular volume depletion in a 24-hour porcine model of intra-abdominal hypertension. J Trauma 2003;55:734–40.

56. Michard F, Alaya S, Zarka V, et al. Global end-diastolic volume as an indicator of cardiac preload in patients with septic shock. Chest 2003;124:1900–8.

57. Michard F, Teboul JL. Predicting fluid responsiveness in ICU patients: a critical analysis of the evidence. Chest 2002;121:2000–8.

58. Simon RJ, Friedlander MH, Ivatury RR, et al. Hemorrhage lowers the threshold for intra-abdominal hypertension-induced pulmonary dysfunction. J Trauma 1997;42: 398–403 [discussion: 4–5].

59. Burchard KW, Ciombor DM, McLeod MK, et al. Positive end expiratory pressure with increased intra-abdominal pressure. Surg Gynecol Obstet 1985;161:313–8.

60. Pelosi P, Ravagnan I, Giurati G, et al. Positive end-expiratory pressure improves respiratory function in obese but not in normal subjects during anesthesia and paralysis. Anesthesiology 1999;91:1221–31.

61. Sugrue M, D'Amours S. The problems with positive end expiratory pressure (PEEP) in association with abdominal compartment syndrome (ACS). J Trauma 2001;51: 419–20.

62. Sussman AM, Boyd CR, Williams JS, et al. Effect of positive end-expiratory pressure on intra-abdominal pressure. South Med J 1991;84:697–700.

63. Cheatham ML, White MW, Sagraves SG, et al. Abdominal perfusion pressure: a superior parameter in the assessment of intra-abdominal hypertension. J Trauma 2000;49:621–6 [discussion: 6–7].

64. Malbrain ML. Abdominal perfusion pressure as a prognostic marker in intra-abdominal hypertension. In: Vincent JL, editor. Yearbook of intensive care and emergency medicine. Berlin: Springer-Verlag; 2002. p. 792–814.

65. Mertens zur Borg IR, Verbrugge SJ, Olvera C. Pathophysiology: respiratory. In: Ivatury R, Cheatham M, Malbrain M, Sugrue M, editors. Abdominal compartment syndrome. Georgetown (TX): Landes Bioscience; 2006. p. 105–18.

66. Ranieri VM, Brienza N, Santostasi S, et al. Impairment of lung and chest wall mechanics in patients with acute respiratory distress syndrome: role of abdominal distension. Am J Respir Crit Care Med 1997;156:1082–91.

67. Gattinoni L, Pelosi P, Suter PM, et al. Acute respiratory distress syndrome caused by pulmonary and extrapulmonary disease. Different syndromes? Am J Respir Crit Care Med 1998;158:3–11.

68. Mutoh T, Lamm WJ, Embree LJ, et al. Abdominal distension alters regional pleural pressures and chest wall mechanics in pigs in vivo. J Appl Physiol 1991;70:2611–8.

69. Mutoh T, Lamm WJ, Embree LJ, et al. Volume infusion produces abdominal distension, lung compression, and chest wall stiffening in pigs. J Appl Physiol 1992;72:575–82.

70. Pelosi P, Quintel M, Malbrain ML. Effect of intra-abdominal pressure on respiratory mechanics. Acta Clin Belg Suppl 2007;62:78–88.

71. Quintel M, Pelosi P, Caironi P, et al. An increase of abdominal pressure increases pulmonary edema in oleic acid-induced lung injury. Am J Respir Crit Care Med 2004;169:534–41.

72. De Keulenaer BL, De Backer A, Schepens DR, et al. Abdominal compartment syndrome related to noninvasive ventilation. Intensive Care Med 2003;29:1177–81.

73. Hering R, Vorwerk R, Wrigge H, et al. Prone positioning, systemic hemodynamics, hepatic indocyanine green kinetics, and gastric intramucosal energy balance in patients with acute lung injury. Intensive Care Med 2002;28:53–8.

74. Hering R, Wrigge H, Vorwerk R, et al. The effects of prone positioning on intraabdominal pressure and cardiovascular and renal function in patients with acute lung injury. Anesth Analg 2001;92:1226–31.

75. De Waele JJ, Benoit D, Hoste E, et al. A role for muscle relaxation in patients with abdominal compartment syndrome? Intensive Care Med 2003;29:332.

76. Diebel LN, Wilson RF, Dulchavsky SA, et al. Effect of increased intra-abdominal pressure on hepatic arterial, portal venous, and hepatic microcirculatory blood flow. J Trauma 1992;33:279–82 [discussion: 82–3].

77. Wendon J, Biancofiore G, Auzinger G. Intra-abdominal hypertension and the liver. In: Ivatury R, Cheatham M, Malbrain M, et al, editors. Abdominal compartment syndrome. Georgetown (TX): Landes Bioscience; 2006. p. 138–43.

78. Biancofiore G, Bindi ML, Boldrini A, et al. Intraabdominal pressure in liver transplant recipients: incidence and clinical significance. Transplant Proc 2004;36:547–9.

79. Biancofiore G, Bindi ML, Romanelli AM, et al. Intra-abdominal pressure monitoring in liver transplant recipients: a prospective study. Intensive Care Med 2003;29:30–6.

80. Michelet P, Roch A, Gainnier M, et al. Influence of support on intra-abdominal pressure, hepatic kinetics of indocyanine green and extravascular lung water during prone positioning in patients with ARDS: a randomized crossover study. Crit Care 2005;9:R251–7.

81. Schein M. Abdominal compartment syndrome: historical background. In: Ivatury R, Cheatham M, Malbrain M, et al, editors. Abdominal compartment syndrome. Georgetown (TX): Landes Bioscience; 2006. p. 1–7.

82. Biancofiore G, Bindi ML, Romanelli AM, et al. Postoperative intra-abdominal pressure and renal function after liver transplantation. Arch Surg 2003;138:703–6.

83. Sugrue M, Hallal A, D'Amours S. Intra-abdominal pressure hypertension and the kidney. In: Ivatury R, Cheatham M, Malbrain M, et al, editors. Abdominal compartment syndrome. Georgetown (TX): Landes Bioscience; 2006. p. 119–28.

84. Sugrue M, Buist MD, Hourihan F, et al. Prospective study of intra-abdominal hypertension and renal function after laparotomy. Br J Surg 1995;82:235–8.

85. Sugrue M, Jones F, Deane SA, et al. Intra-abdominal hypertension is an independent cause of postoperative renal impairment. Arch Surg 1999;134:1082–5.

86. Kirkpatrick AW, Colistro R, Laupland KB, et al. Renal arterial resistive index response to intraabdominal hypertension in a porcine model. Crit Care Med 2006;35(1):207–13.

87. Bradley SE, Mudge GH, Blake WD, et al. The effect of increased intra-abdominal pressure on the renal excretion of water and electrolytes in normal human subjects and in patients with diabetes insipidus. Acta Clin Belg 1955;10:209–23.

88. Harman PK, Kron IL, McLachlan HD, et al. Elevated intra-abdominal pressure and renal function. Ann Surg 1982;196:594–7.

89. Kron IL, Harman PK, Nolan SP. The measurement of intra-abdominal pressure as a criterion for abdominal re-exploration. Ann Surg 1984;199:28–30.

90. Luca A, Feu F, Garcia-Pagan JC, et al. Favorable effects of total paracentesis on splanchnic hemodynamics in cirrhotic patients with tense ascites. Hepatology 1994;20:30–3.

91. Jacques T, Lee R. Improvement of renal function after relief of raised intra-abdominal pressure due to traumatic retroperitoneal haematoma. Anaesth Intensive Care 1988;16:478–82.

92. Morris JA Jr, Eddy VA, Blinman TA, et al. The staged celiotomy for trauma. Issues in unpacking and reconstruction. Ann Surg 1993;217:576–84.

93. Shelly MP, Robinson AA, Hesford JW, et al. Haemodynamic effects following surgical release of increased intra-abdominal pressure. Br J Anaesth 1987;59:800–5.

94. Cullen DJ, Coyle JP, Teplick R, et al. Cardiovascular, pulmonary, and renal effects of massively increased intra-abdominal pressure in critically ill patients. Crit Care Med 1989;17:118–21.

95. Smith JH, Merrell RC, Raffin TA. Reversal of postoperative anuria by decompressive celiotomy. Arch Intern Med 1985;145:553–4.

96. Richards WO, Scovill W, Shin B, et al. Acute renal failure associated with increased intra-abdominal pressure. Ann Surg 1983;197:183–7.

97. Stothert JC. Evaluation of decapsulation of the canine kidney on renal function following acute ischemia. J Surg Res 1979;26:560–4.

98. Gewertz BL, Krupski W, Wheeler HT, et al. Effect of renal decapsulation on cortical hemodynamics in the postischemic kidney. J Surg Res 1980;28:252–9.

99. Ivatury R, Diebel L. Intra-abdominal hypertension and the splanchnic bed. In: Ivatury R, Cheatham M, Malbrain M, et al, editors. Abdominal compartment syndrome. Georgetown (TX): Landes Bioscience; 2006. p. 129–37.

100. Diebel LN, Dulchavsky SA, Brown WJ. Splanchnic ischemia and bacterial translocation in the abdominal compartment syndrome. J Trauma 1997;43:852–5.

101. Diebel LN, Dulchavsky SA, Wilson RF. Effect of increased intra-abdominal pressure on mesenteric arterial and intestinal mucosal blood flow. J Trauma1992; 33:45–8 [discussion: 8–9].

102. Balogh Z, Moore FA. Postinjury secondary abdominal compartment syndrome. In: Ivatury R, Cheatham M, Malbrain M, et al, editors. Abdominal compartment syndrome. Georgetown (TX): Landes Bioscience; 2006. p. 170–7.

103. Raeburn CD, Moore EE. Abdominal compartment syndrome provokes multiple organ failure: animal and human supporting evidence. In: Ivatury R, Cheatham M, Malbrain M, et al, editors. Abdominal compartment syndrome. Georgetown (TX): Landes Bioscience; 2006. p. 157–69.

104. Sugrue M, Jones F, Lee A, et al. Intraabdominal pressure and gastric intramucosal pH: is there an association? World J Surg 1996;20:988–91.

105. Ivatury RR, Porter JM, Simon RJ, et al. Intra-abdominal hypertension after life-threatening penetrating abdominal trauma: prophylaxis, incidence, and clinical relevance to gastric mucosal pH and abdominal compartment syndrome. J Trauma 1998;44:1016–21 [discussion: 21–3].

106. Balogh Z, McKinley BA, Cocanour CS, et al. Supranormal trauma resuscitation causes more cases of abdominal compartment syndrome. 2003;138:637–42 [discussion: 42–3].

107. Balogh Z, McKinley BA, Cox CS Jr, et al. Abdominal compartment syndrome: the cause or effect of postinjury multiple organ failure. Shock 2003;20:483–92.

108. Moore FA. The role of the gastrointestinal tract in postinjury multiple organ failure. Am J Surg 1999;178:449–53.

109. Eleftheriadis E, Kotzampassi K, Papanotas K, et al. Gut ischemia, oxidative stress, and bacterial translocation in elevated abdominal pressure in rats. World J Surg 1996;20:11–6.

110. Diebel L, Saxe J, Dulchavsky S. Effect of intra-abdominal pressure on abdominal wall blood flow. Am Surg 1992;58:573–5.

111. Wesley JR, Drongowski R, Coran AG. Intragastric pressure measurement: a guide for reduction and closure of the silastic chimney in omphalocele and gastroschisis. J Pediatr Surg 1981;16:264–70.

112. Rizzo A, Davis PC, Hamm CR, et al. Intraoperative vesical pressure measurements as a guide in the closure of abdominal wall defects. Am Surg 1996;62:192–6.

113. Kuhn MA, Tuggle DW. Abdominal compartment syndrome in the pediatric patient. In: Ivatury R, Cheatham M, Malbrain M, et al, editors. Abdominal compartment syndrome. Georgetown (TX): Landes Bioscience; 2006. p. 217–22.

114. Ivy ME. Secondary abdominal compartment syndrome in burns. In: Ivatury R, Cheatham M, Malbrain M, et al, editors. Abdominal compartment syndrome. Georgetown (TX): Landes Bioscience; 2006;178–86.

115. Demling RH, Crawford G, Lind L, et al. Restrictive pulmonary dysfunction caused by the grafted chest and abdominal burn. Crit Care Med 1988;16:743–7.

116. Greenhalgh DG, Warden GD. The importance of intra-abdominal pressure measurements in burned children. J Trauma 1994;36:685–90.

117. Hobson KG, Young KM, Ciraulo A, et al. Release of abdominal compartment syndrome improves survival in patients with burn injury. J Trauma 2002;53:1129–33.

118. Ivy ME, Atweh NA, Palmer J, et al. Intra-abdominal hypertension and abdominal compartment syndrome in burn patients. J Trauma 2000;49:387–91.

119. Ivy ME, Possenti PP, Kepros J, et al. Abdominal compartment syndrome in patients with burns. J Burn Care Rehabil 1999;20:351–3.

120. Latenser BA, Kowal-Vern A, Kimball D, et al. A pilot study comparing percutaneous decompression with decompressive laparotomy for acute abdominal compartment syndrome in thermal injury. J Burn Care Rehabil 2002;23:190–5.

121. Ziakas PD, Voulgarelis M, Felekouras E, et al. Myelofibrosis-associated massive splenomegaly: a cause of increased intra-abdominal pressure, pulmonary hypertension, and positional dyspnea. Am J Hematol 2005;80:128–32.

122. Hamad GG, Peitzman AB. Morbid obesity and chronic intra-abdominal hypertension. In: Ivatury R, Cheatham M, Malbrain M, et al, editors. Abdominal compartment syndrome. Georgetown (TX): Landes Bioscience; 2006. p. 187–94.

123. Sugerman HJ. Increased intra-abdominal pressure in obesity. Int J Obes Relat Metab Disord 1998;22:1138.

124. Ueland K, Novy MJ, Peterson EN, et al. Maternal cardiovascular dynamics. IV. The influence of gestational age on the maternal cardiovascular response to posture and exercise. Am J Obstet Gynecol 1969;104:856–64.

125. Lemaire BM, van Erp WF. Laparoscopic surgery during pregnancy. Surg Endosc 1997;11:15–8.

126. O'Rourke N, Kodali BS. Laparoscopic surgery during pregnancy. Curr Opin Anaesthesiol 2006;19:254–9.

127. Scalea TM, Bochicchio GV, Habashi N, et al. Increased intra-abdominal, intrathoracic, and intracranial pressure after severe brain injury: multiple compartment syndrome. J Trauma 2007;62:647–56.

128. De laet I, Citerio G, Malbrain ML. The influence of intraabdominal hypertension on the central nervous system: current insights and clinical recommendations, is it all in the head? Acta Clin Belg Suppl 2007;62:89–97.

129. Malbrain ML, Wilmer A. The polycompartment syndrome: towards an understanding of the interactions between different compartments! Intensive Care Med 2007;33:1869–72.

130. De laet IE, De Waele JJ, Malbrain MLNG. Fluid resuscitation and intra-abdominal hypertension. In: Vincent J-L, editor. Yearbook of intensive care and emergency medicine. Berlin: Springer-Verlag; 2008. p. 536–48.

131. Kirkpatrick AW, De Waele JJ, Ball CG, et al. The secondary and recurrent abdominal compartment syndrome. Acta Clin Belg Suppl 2007;62:60–5.

132. Maxwell RA, Fabian TC, Croce MA, et al. Secondary abdominal compartment syndrome: an underappreciated manifestation of severe hemorrhagic shock. J Trauma 1999;47:995–9.

133. Balogh Z, McKinley BA, Cocanour CS, et al. Secondary abdominal compartment syndrome is an elusive early complication of traumatic shock resuscitation. Am J Surg 2002;184:538–43 [discussion: 43–4].

134. Alsous F, Khamiees M, DeGirolamo A, et al. Negative fluid balance predicts survival in patients with septic shock: a retrospective pilot study. Chest 2000;117:1749–54.

135. Daugherty EL, Hongyan L, Taichman D, et al. Abdominal compartment syndrome is common in medical intensive care unit patients receiving large-volume resuscitation. J Intensive Care Med 2007;22:294–9.

136. Morishita Y, Harada T, Moriyama Y, et al. Simultaneous retrieval of the heart and liver from a single donor: an evaluation through preservation and transplantation. J Heart Transplant 1988;7:269–73.

137. Tyagi S, Kaul UA, Nair M, et al. Balloon angioplasty of the aorta in Takayasu's arteritis: initial and long-term results. Am Heart J 1992;124:876–82.

138. Oda J, Ueyama M, Yamashita K, et al. Hypertonic lactated saline resuscitation reduces the risk of abdominal compartment syndrome in severely burned patients. J Trauma 2006;60:64–71.

139. O'Mara MS, Slater H, Goldfarb IW, et al. A prospective, randomized evaluation of intra-abdominal pressures with crystalloid and colloid resuscitation in burn patients. J Trauma 2005;58:1011–8.
140. Reintam A, Parm P, Kitus R, et al. Primary and secondary intra-abdominal hypertension— different impact on ICU outcome. Intensive Care Med 2008;34(9):1624–31.
141. Vidal M, Ruiz Weisser J, Gonzalez F, et al. Incidence and clinical effects of intraabdominal hypertension in critically ill patients. Crit Care Med 2008;36(6):1823–31.
142. Malbrain ML, De Laet I. AIDS is coming to your ICU: be prepared for acute bowel injury and acute intestinal distress syndrome. Intensive Care Med 2008;34(9):1565–9.
143. Kimball EJ. Intra-abdominal hypertension and the abdominal compartment syndrome: 'ARDS' of the gut. Int J Intensive Care 2006;1–7.
144. De Laet IE, Hoste EA, De Waele JJ. Survey on the perception and management of the abdominal compartment syndrome among Belgian surgeons. Acta Chir Belg 2007;107:648–52.
145. Kirkpatrick AW, Balogh Z, Ball CG, et al. The secondary abdominal compartment syndrome: iatrogenic or unavoidable? J Am Coll Surg 2006;202:668–79.
146. Mayberry JC. Prevention of abdominal compartment syndrome. In: Ivatury R, Cheatham M, Malbrain M, et al, editors. Abdominal compartment syndrome. Georgetown (TX): Landes Bioscience; 2006. p. 221–9.
147. Parr M, Olvera C. Medical management of abdominal compartment syndrome. In: Ivatury R, Cheatham M, Malbrain M, et al, editors. Abdominal compartment syndrome. Georgetown (TX): Landes Bioscience; 2006. p. 230–7.
148. Macalino JU, Goldman RK, Mayberry JC. Medical management of abdominal compartment syndrome: case report and a caution. Asian J Surg 2002;25:244–6.
149. Kimball EJ, Mone M. Influence of neuromuscular blockade on intra-abdominal pressure. Crit Care Med 2005;33:A38.
150. Kimball WR, Loring SH, Basta SJ, et al. Effects of paralysis with pancuronium on chest wall statics in awake humans. J Appl Physiol 1985;58:1638–45.
151. Drummond GB, Duncan MK. Abdominal pressure during laparoscopy: effects of fentanyl. Br J Anaesth 2002;88:384–8.
152. Voss M, Pinheiro J, Reynolds J, et al. Endoscopic components separation for abdominal compartment syndrome. Am J Surg 2003;186:158–63.
153. Bauer JJ, Gelernt IM, Salky BA, et al. Is routine postoperative nasogastric decompression really necessary? Ann Surg 1985;201:233–6.
154. Cheatham ML, Chapman WC, Key SP, et al. A meta-analysis of selective versus routine nasogastric decompression after elective laparotomy. Ann Surg 1995;221:469–76.
155. Moss G, Friedman RC. Abdominal decompression: increased efficency by esophageal aspiration utilizing a new nasogastric tube. Am J Surg 1977;133:225–8.
156. Savassi-Rocha PR, Conceicao SA, Ferreira JT, et al. Evaluation of the routine use of the nasogastric tube in digestive operation by a prospective controlled study. Surg Gynecol Obstet 1992;174:317–20.
157. Ponec RJ, Saunders MD, Kimmey MB. Neostigmine for the treatment of acute colonic pseudo-obstruction. N Engl J Med 1999;341:137–41.
158. Wilmer A, Dits H, Malbrain ML, et al. Gastric emptying in the critically ill—the way forward. Intensive Care Med 1997;23:928–9.
159. Madl C, Druml W. Gastrointestinal disorders of the critically ill. Systemic consequences of ileus. Best Pract Res Clin Gastroenterol 2003;17:445–56.

160. Malbrain ML. Abdominal pressure in the critically ill. Curr Opin Crit Care 2000;6: 17–29.
161. Gorecki PJ, Kessler E, Schein M. Abdominal compartment syndrome from intractable constipation. J Am Coll Surg 2000;190:371.
162. van der Spoel JI, Oudemans-van Straaten HM, Stoutenbeek CP, et al. Neostigmine resolves critical illness-related colonic ileus in intensive care patients with multiple organ failure—a prospective, double-blind, placebo-controlled trial. Intensive Care Med 2001;27:822–7.
163. Sugrue M. Abdominal compartment syndrome. Curr Opin Crit Care 2005;11:333–8.
164. Corcos AC, Sherman HF. Percutaneous treatment of secondary abdominal compartment syndrome. J Trauma 2001;51:1062–4.
165. Cabrera J, Falcon L, Gorriz E, et al. Abdominal decompression plays a major role in early postparacentesis haemodynamic changes in cirrhotic patients with tense ascites. Gut 2001;48:384–9.
166. Reckard JM, Chung MH, Varma MK, et al. Management of intraabdominal hypertension by percutaneous catheter drainage. J Vasc Interv Radiol 2005;16:1019–21.
167. Escorsell A, Gines A, Llach J, et al. Increasing intra-abdominal pressure increases pressure, volume, and wall tension in esophageal varices. Hepatology 2002;36: 936–40.
168. Gotlieb WH, Feldman B, Feldman-Moran O, et al. Intraperitoneal pressures and clinical parameters of total paracentesis for palliation of symptomatic ascites in ovarian cancer. Gynecol Oncol 1998;71:381–5.
169. Navarro-Rodriguez T, Hashimoto CL, Carrilho FJ, et al. Reduction of abdominal pressure in patients with ascites reduces gastroesophageal reflux. Dis Esophagus 2003;16:77–82.
170. Friedlander MH, Simon RJ, Ivatury R, et al. Effect of hemorrhage on superior mesenteric artery flow during increased intra-abdominal pressures. J Trauma 1998; 45:433–89.
171. Gargiulo NJ 3rd, Simon RJ, Leon W, et al. Hemorrhage exacerbates bacterial translocation at low levels of intra-abdominal pressure. Arch Surg 1998;133: 1351–5.
172. Agusti M, Elizalde JI, Adalia R, et al. Dobutamine restores intestinal mucosal blood flow in a porcine model of intra-abdominal hyperpressure. Crit Care Med 2000;28: 467–72.
173. Oda S, Hirasawa H, Shiga H, et al. Management of intra-abdominal hypertension in patients with severe acute pancreatitis with continuous hemodiafiltration using a polymethyl methacrylate membrane hemofilter. Ther Apher Dial 2005;9:355–61.
174. Kula R, Szturz P, Sklienka P, et al. A role for negative fluid balance in septic patients with abdominal compartment syndrome? Intensive Care Med 2004;30:2138–9.
175. Vachharajani V, Scott LK, Grier L, et al. Medical management of severe intraabdominal hypertension with aggressive diuresis and continuous ultra-filtration. Internet J Emerg Intensive Care Med. Available at: http://www.ispub.com/ostia/index.phpxmlFilePath=journals/ijeicm/vol6n2/ultr. Accessed March 5, 2012.
176. Valenza F, Irace M, Guglielmi M, et al. Effects of continuous negative extraabdominal pressure on cardiorespiratory function during abdominal hypertension: an experimental study. Intensive Care Med 2005;31:105–11.
177. Valenza F, Bottino N, Canavesi K, et al. Intra-abdominal pressure may be decreased non-invasively by continuous negative extra-abdominal pressure (NEXAP). Intensive Care Med 2003;29:2063–7.

178. Valenza F, Gattinoni L. Continuous negative abdominal pressure. In: Ivatury R, Cheatham M, Malbrain M, et al, editors. Abdominal compartment syndrome. Georgetown (TX): Landes Bioscience; 2006. p. 238–51.

179. Kacmaz A, Polat A, User Y, et al. Octreotide improves reperfusion-induced oxidative injury in acute abdominal hypertension in rats. J Gastrointest Surg 2004;8:113–9.

180. Sener G, Kacmaz A, User Y, et al. Melatonin ameliorates oxidative organ damage induced by acute intra-abdominal compartment syndrome in rats. J Pineal Res 2003;35:163–8.

181. Mertens zur Borg IR, Verbrugge SJ, Kolkman KA. Anesthetic considerations in abdominal compartment syndrome. In: Ivatury R, Cheatham M, Malbrain M, et al, editors. Abdominal compartment syndrome. Georgetown (TX): Landes Bioscience; 2006;252–63.

182. Balogh Z, Moore FA, Goettler CE, et al. Management of abdominal compartment syndrome. In: Ivatury R, Cheatham M, Malbrain M, et al, editors. Abdominal compartment syndrome. Georgetown (TX): Landes Bioscience; 2006. p. 264–94.

183. De Laet IE, Ravyts M, Vidts W, et al. Current insights in intra-abdominal hypertension and abdominal compartment syndrome: open the abdomen and keep it open!. Langenbecks Arch Surg 2008;393:833–47.

184. Cheatham ML, Safcsak K, Llerena LE, et al. Long-term physical, mental, and functional consequences of abdominal decompression. 2004;56:237–41 [discussion: 41–2].

185. Kimball EJ, Kim W, Cheatham ML, et al. Clinical awareness of intra-abdominal hypertension and abdominal compartment syndrome in 2007. Acta Clin Belg 2007;62(Suppl):66–73.

186. Burch JM, Moore EE, Moore FA, et al. The abdominal compartment syndrome. Surg Clin North Am 1996;76:833–42.

187. Ivatury RR, Sugerman HJ, Peitzman AB. Abdominal compartment syndrome: recognition and management. Adv Surg 2001;35:251–69.

Reconstruction of the Foot After Leg or Foot Compartment Syndrome

Mark D. Perry, MD[a],*, Arthur Manoli II, MD[b]

KEYWORDS

• Early foot repair • Late foot repair • Deformity • Compartment syndrome

KEY POINTS

- Compartment syndrome should be treated early and aggressively to prevent late complications.
- Patients may have late deformity because of a failure of diagnosis, inadequate decompression, or a delay in fasciotomies. Late reconstruction will allow a plantigrade and relatively functional foot.
- Complete excision of scarred muscle will prevent recurrence in established deformities.
- Early treatment may prevent significant functional impairment by well placed tenotomies. In patients with severe long-term deformities with extensive soft tissue contraction, incremental correction may be an appropriate intermediate intervention.

Compartment syndrome has been well recognized as a complication of lower extremity injury. Nevertheless, literature discussing specific reconstructions for compartment syndrome sequelae is scarce.[1,2] Seddon[3] in 1966 described the pathophysiology of lower limb contractures secondary to compartment syndrome, and Manoli and coworkers in 1991 presented their work on the treatment of established ischemic contractures.[2]

The pathophysiology of compartment syndrome is well understood. Interestingly, upper limb ischemic contracture occurs owing to a different mechanism than lower limb injury. Compartment syndrome in the upper limb tends to develop from a vascular insult of the brachial artery, which results in predictable ischemia distally.[3]

A version of this article was previously published in *Foot and Ankle Clinics* 11:1.
The authors do not have any commercial or proprietary interest in any equipment mentioned in this article.
[a] Department of Orthopaedic Surgery, University of Texas Southwestern Medical Center, 5323 Harry Hines Boulevard, Dallas, TX 75390-8883, USA; [b] Michigan International Foot and Ankle Center, 44555 Woodward Avenue, Suite 105, Pontiac, MI 48341, USA
* Corresponding author.
E-mail address: Mark.Perry@UTSouthwestern.edu

Crit Care Nurs Clin N Am 24 (2012) 311–322
doi:10.1016/j.ccell.2012.03.005
0899-5885/12/$ – see front matter © 2012 Elsevier Inc. All rights reserved.

Lower limb compartment syndrome is often associated with a fracture or a crush type injury. These tissues experience not only ischemia from increased compartment pressures but also a direct crush injury resulting in cellular damage.[4] Elevation ischemia intraoperatively or from high postoperative leg elevation is an increasing cause of compartment syndrome.

PREVENTION

Despite the increasing vigilance in the orthopedic community to diagnosis compartment syndrome, it is still an often preventable but dreaded complication.[5] Compartment syndrome must be recognized and "fixed" by treating it acutely. Avoidance of the problem leads to catastrophic late complications. The physician must perform an honest assessment evaluating the empirical and clinical evidence.[6] Denial of compartment syndrome is never appropriate treatment.

Polytrauma patients see multiple physicians[7] who subsequently run many tests[8] and perform multiple evaluations,[9] increasing the chance of failed communication resulting in a critical delay in diagnosis. Failing to make a diagnosis of compartment syndrome is the most common treatment error.[10,11] Clinical judgment unfortunately is inaccurate, and only dramatic compartment syndromes are easily evident. The "subtle" compartment syndromes are the most difficult to define, resulting in significant deformities and late complications.

The diagnosis of compartment syndrome should be suspected in many clinical settings.[12–18] Orthopedic surgeons should have a high degree of suspicion when treating fractures of the tibial shaft and tibial plateau, high-energy ankle injuries, and pilon fractures. Fractures of the femur and the foot can also result in compartment syndrome. Knee dislocations and vascular bypass surgery can result in compartment syndrome from prolonged vascular compromise and reperfusion. Transplant surgery and cardiac bypass surgery can cause compartment syndrome from prolonged hypotension. Infections and circumferential burns are also known to provide increased compartment pressures. Drug overdose and prolonged pressure can cause compartment syndromes in unusual locations. Prolonged limb elevation during urologic, general, transplant, and orthopedic surgery can result in muscle damage and compartment syndrome during reperfusion. Unusual conditions causing compartment syndrome include hemophilia and snake bites.

Leg compartment syndrome late sequelae occur secondary to a delay in diagnosis or to inadequate decompression. Orthopedic surgeons and general surgeons can treat acute compartment syndrome of the leg. Depending on the training of the surgeon, the release may be inadequate. **Fig. 1** shows the leg of a patient whose fasciotomy performed by a nonorthopedic service for compartment syndrome was done too high, missing the posterior compartment. The deep posterior compartment was never released, resulting in a severe deformity; however, the patient achieved a plantigrade foot with relatively good function following scarred muscle excision and a midfoot osteotomy.

Fig. 2 illustrates another error during fasciotomies. Although the compartments were released, the skin bridge anteriorly was too small and necrosed. Subsequently, the patient's large anterior wound prevented internal fixation of his bimalleolar ankle fracture.

Orthopedic surgeons focus on long skin incisions with direct visualization of the fascia releasing between the intermuscular septae. In addition, four compartment fasciotomies should be performed if lower limb compartment syndrome is suspected in a trauma situation. A two-compartment release is appropriate only for nontraumatic, chronic exertional compartment syndrome situations.

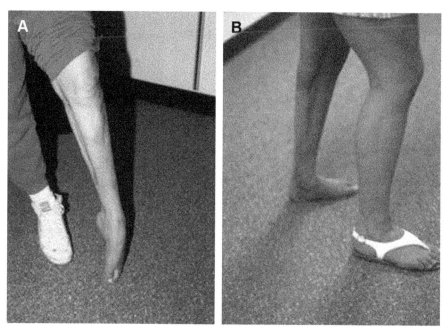

Fig. 1. (*A*) Preoperative and (*B*) postoperative clinical photographs of an untreated deep posterior compartment syndrome. A plantigrade foot was attainable following scarred muscle excision and a midfoot osteotomy.

Isolated foot compartment syndromes have been described. Late complications include contracture of the quadratus plantae.[19,20] Approximately 10% of intra-articular calcaneal fractures develop foot compartment syndrome.[21] Foot compartment syndrome can also occur after Lisfranc fracture-dislocations, crush injuries, elevation ischemia, and multiple metatarsal fractures. Any time there is a combination of forefoot, midfoot, and hindfoot injury, foot compartment syndrome must be suspected.[22–24]

The late foot deficit after foot compartment syndrome includes stiffness and decreased sensation. The lesser toes develop clawing owing to intrinsic muscle weakness or contracture, which can be significantly painful. Foot compartments

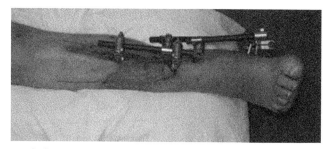

Fig. 2. Photograph demonstrates skin necrosis treated with a split-thickness skin graft after fasciotomy wounds were placed incorrectly.

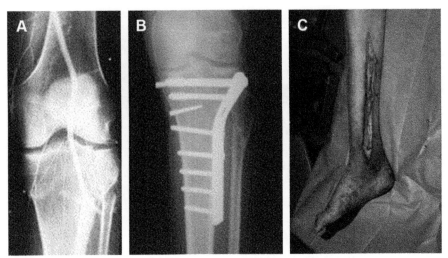

Fig. 3. (A) Angiogram showing lateral tibial plateau fracture. (B) Internal fixation. (C) After multiple débridements, the wound became infected and eventually required a below knee amputation.

connect between the calcaneal compartment and the deep posterior compartment of the leg.[25,26] Foot compartments should be released to prevent the development of leg compartment syndrome.[26] Some physicians argue that isolated acute foot compartment syndrome should be observed and a late reconstruction performed if necessary.

DELAY IN DIAGNOSIS IN THE ACUTE PHASE OF CARE

Patients may present late in the acute phase after the pain has become reduced, indicating the muscle is no longer viable. This "gray area" exists for patients outside of 6 hours of symptoms. If there is an opportunity to prevent compartment syndrome from developing in other compartments, a fasciotomy must be performed. Exposed dead muscle may become infected, potentially leading to below knee amputation despite multiple débridements (**Fig. 3**).

In patients for whom there is no expectation of salvaging viable muscle after a compartment syndrome, fasciotomy should not be performed. The muscle necrosis will not progress to infection[27] if the skin is intact. If necessary, the patient can be placed temporarily on dialysis during the rhabdomyolysis and the resulting deformity addressed later.

LATE TECHNIQUES

Clinically, the diagnosis of deep posterior compartment fibrosis is established by the presence of equinus and cavus with a resulting heel varus and claw toes.[25,28] The goal of reconstruction of the foot is to restore a functional and minimally painful plantigrade foot. The contracture is treated once the deforming forces and scarred muscles have been studied. All fibrotic muscle must be released and excised, because incomplete excision will cause recurrence.

Although rare, an amputation may be indicated because of pain, ulceration, and rigid deformity. **Fig. 4** shows the dorsum of the foot of a patient with a closed head injury, a spinal cord injury, and leg compartment syndrome. At the time of presentation, wounds

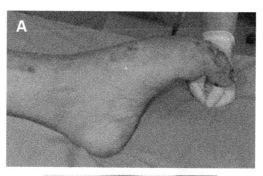

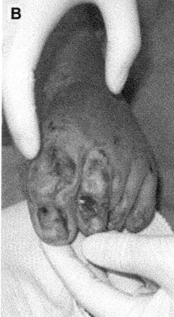

Fig. 4. Toe ulcers. (*A*) Lateral and (*B*) anteroposterior photographs following nontreatment of post compartment syndrome deformity.

had developed after the patient was pushed in a wheel chair with the ankle in a rigid plantar flexed position. This case illustrates the importance of a neutral ankle position, even in nonambulatory patients. In these patients, the limb can be salvaged by appropriate releases or transfers, preserving patient body image, acting as a counterweight for wheelchair sitting, and assisting in transfers.

Although compartment syndrome can affect all compartments, the resulting deformity depends on the degree of involvement and the anatomy of the muscles affected. Although an anterior compartment syndrome may result in loss of active ankle dorsiflexion, this may not cause a functional deformity. Passive stretching during sleep may maintain motion. An isolated posterior compartment syndrome involving the flexor hallucis longus (FHL) or posterior tibial tendon may cause a significant deformity owing to a lack of antagonistic muscle contraction and strength of the anterior compartment.

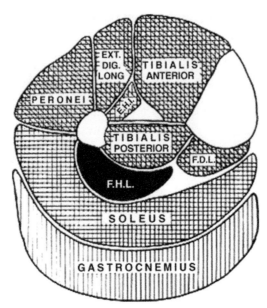

Fig. 5. Diagram showing vulnerability to ischemia of muscles of the leg. The flexor hallucis longus is the most frequently damaged, but the interior muscles, which are superficial, suffer considerably. (*From* Seddon HJ. Volkmann's ischaemia in the lower limb. J Bone Joint Surg Br 1966;48(4):627–36; with permission.) © British Editorial Society of Bone and Joint Surgery.

The posterior compartment is the most likely to cause late symptoms (**Fig. 5**). Over 60% of Seddon's subjects had FHL involvement, with the tibialis posterior and the flexor digitorum longus having 40% involvement. In contrast, the gastrocnemius (20%) and the soleus (25%) were less affected.[3]

Fig. 6 shows the leg of an intensive care unit patient in whom systemic inflammatory response syndrome (SIRS) and compartment syndrome developed. Releases

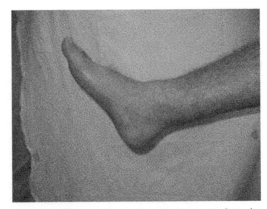

Fig. 6. A deformity of plantar flexion without inversion occurs when the deep compartment is spared.

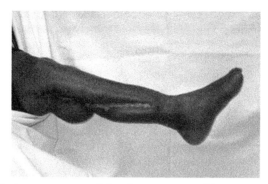

Fig. 7. Photograph shows recurrence following tenotomy without scarred muscle excision.

were performed, and 6 months later, the patient still had residual deformity. The ankle was fixed in 20 degrees of plantar flexion without varus position of the foot. The calf was rigid to palpation. The patient developed fibrosis of the soleus muscle, without involvement of the deep posterior compartment.

Contracture of the deep posterior compartment causes the typical late appearance of leg compartment syndrome. The foot is held internally rotated and in a cavus position with the heel in corresponding varus. Release of the Achilles tendon alone will not correct this deformity; instead, the ischemic muscle should be excised to correct the foot position and prevent recurrence.

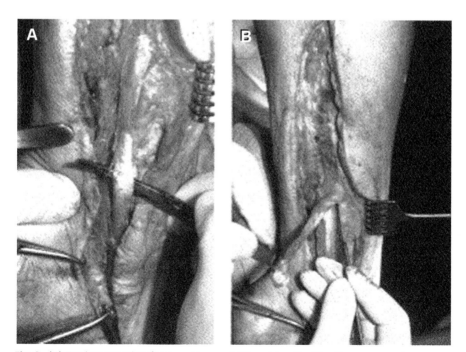

Fig. 8. (*A*) Testing a tendon for excursion and (*B*) excising the fibrotic components.

Fig. 7 demonstrates the recurrence of deformity after tenotomy treatment. This 47-year-old woman developed compartment syndrome as a complication of a vascular procedure. Despite acute fasciotomies, late deformity developed. In the operating room, it was determined that a posterior release of the Achilles tendon resolved all but 10 degrees of plantar flexion. A tenotomy of the posterior tibial tendon was also performed to place the ankle in a neutral position. Despite postoperative placement in an ankle foot orthosis, after 16 months, a rigid equinus deformity recurred.

Patients with a cavus foot secondary to compartment syndrome also present with a significant internal rotation of the foot and a varus heel. The patient will correct this deformity by externally rotating at the hip. Some of the patients in the study by Manoli and coworkers[2] were previously recommended to undergo rotational osteotomies of this deformity because of the believed internal rotation of the fracture at the deformity site.

Occasionally, an early release of the claw toes via tenotomy may be performed to prevent further development of deformity. A heel cord lengthening or slide may prevent a major equinus component from developing. During late surgical reconstruction, muscle excision, release of contracted joint capsules and tissue, as well as osteotomies and fusions may be required to achieve a plantigrade foot.[29]

Exploration of the compartments requires good visualization. Each tendon must be checked for excursion individually (**Fig. 8**). Any tendon without excursion must have all nonviable muscle removed. A first metatarsal osteotomy and a calcaneal osteotomy can correct heel varus.[30]

Claw toes that develop from foot compartment syndrome may require proximal interphalangeal (PIP) joint resections (**Fig. 9**). The contracted flexor tendon may lack excursion, preventing a functional flexor to extensor tendon transfer.[29] If flexible but

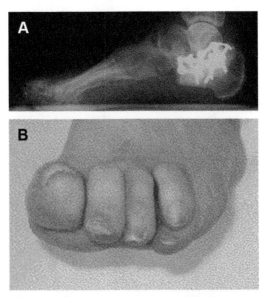

Fig. 9. (*A*) A displaced intra-articular calcaneal fracture that did not undergo fasciotomy for foot compartment syndrome. (*B*) Rigid claw toes that subsequently developed.

tight, the flexor tendon should be taken as far distal to the PIP as possible to have enough length to transfer to the base of the proximal phalanx.

Following débridement of ischemic muscle, the surgical wounds are closed over a drain to prevent hematoma.[2] These limbs have undergone significant trauma, and

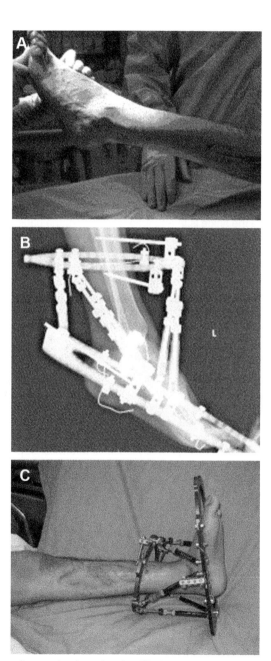

Fig. 10. (*A*) Preoperative maximal passive dorsiflexion. (*B*) Application of frame. (*C*) Correction after incremental changes over 2 months.

skin problems can occur after late reconstructions. Great care needs to be taken in handling the soft tissue envelope during reconstruction. Patients are kept in a cast and encouraged to weight bear as tolerated. Casting holds the ankle in a neutral position during recovery. If bony work such as subtalar fusion, triple arthrodesis, or osteotomy has been performed, weight bearing should be delayed while the ankle is splinted. Early weight bearing will assist dorsiflexion.

In situations where a tremendous deformity exits, or in a setting of a poor tissue envelope, initial correction may be achieved with an external frame (**Fig. 10**). A percutaneous tendo-Achilles lengthening and incremental adjustment will allow the foot to be placed under the leg with minimal surgical morbidity. At the authors' center, a multiplanar frame has been used to correct ischemic contractures 1 and 2 years post injury. The frame concurrently corrects the plantar flexion and the varus deformity. Current results for a patient at 1 year and for another at 6 months postoperatively have revealed no deformity or recurrence. External fixation was continued for 3 months following deformity correction. Once the foot was in a position allowing weight bearing (plantar flexion of approximately 20 degrees), a custom footplate was attached to the frame. Lymphedema may occur during the deformity correction secondary to compression of the sinus tarsi. If lymphedema suddenly develops, the frame is adjusted to relax the deformity, and the desired position is achieved at a slower rate. In these cases, once the ankle is in a functional position, the patient may be followed clinically and, if necessary, undergo scarred muscle excision in a standard fashion if the deformity starts to recur.

Recurrence is minimized by excising scarred muscle as well as the tendon components. Hansen's group did not find pes planus after posterior tibial excision.[2] The spring ligament should not be disrupted. All viable muscle is kept and may be used for tendon transfers. Clawson's test of the long flexors may not be possible in patients with leg compartment syndrome because of ankle stiffness.[31]

SUMMARY

Compartment syndrome should be treated early and aggressively to prevent late complications. Patients may have late deformity because of a failure of diagnosis, inadequate decompression, or a delay in fasciotomies.[32] Late reconstruction will allow a plantigrade and relatively functional foot. Complete excision of scarred muscle will prevent recurrence in established deformities. Early treatment may prevent significant functional impairment by well-placed tenotomies. In patients with severe long-term deformities with extensive soft tissue contraction, incremental correction may be an appropriate intermediate intervention.

REFERENCES

1. Santi MD, Botte MJ. Volkmann's ischemic contracture of the foot and ankle: evaluation and treatment of established deformity. Foot Ankle Int 1995;16(6):368–77.
2. Manoli A 2nd, Smith DG, Hansen ST Jr, Scarred muscle excision for the treatment of established ischemic contracture of the lower extremity. Clin Orthop 1993;292: 309–14.
3. Seddon HJ. Volkmann's ischaemia in the lower limb. J Bone Joint Surg Br 1966;48(4): 627–36.
4. Kikuchi S, Hasue M, Watanabe M. Ischemic contracture in the lower limb. Clin Orthop 1978;134:185–92.
5. Bhattacharyya T, Vrahas MS. The medical-legal aspects of compartment syndrome. J Bone Joint Surg Am 2004;86(4):864–8.

6. Holden CE. Compartmental syndromes following trauma. Clin Orthop 1975;113:95–102.

7. Giannoudis PV, Nicolopoulos C, Dinopoulos H, et al. The impact of lower leg compartment syndrome on health related quality of life. Injury 2002;33(2):117–21.

8. Farrell CM, Rubin DI, Haidukewych GJ. Acute compartment syndrome of the leg following diagnostic electromyography. Muscle Nerve 2003;27(3):374–7.

9. Cascio BM, Wilckens JH, Ain MC, et al. Documentation of acute compartment syndrome at an academic health-care center. J Bone Joint Surg Am 2005;87(2):346–50.

10. Richards H, Langston A, Kulkarni R, et al. Does patient controlled analgesia delay the diagnosis of compartment syndrome following intramedullary nailing of the tibia?. Injury 2004;35(3):296–8.

11. Hope MJ, McQueen MM. Acute compartment syndrome in the absence of fracture. J Orthop Trauma 2004;18(4):220–4.

12. Ashworth MJ, Patel N. Compartment syndrome following ankle fracture-dislocation: a case report. J Orthop Trauma 1998;12(1):67–8.

13. Dhawan A, Doukas WC. Acute compartment syndrome of the foot following an inversion injury of the ankle with disruption of the anterior tibial artery: a case report. J Bone Joint Surg Am 2003;85(3):528–32.

14. Russell GV Jr, Pearsall AW, Caylor MT, et al. Acute compartment syndrome after rupture of the medial head of the gastrocnemius muscle. South Med J 2000;93(2):247–9.

15. Reuben A, Clouting E. Compartment syndrome after thrombolysis for acute myocardial infarction. Emerg Med J 2005;22(1):77.

16. Meldrum R, Lipscomb P. Compartment syndrome of the leg after less than 4 hours of elevation on a fracture table. South Med J 2002; 95(2):269–71.

17. Noorpuri BS, Shahane SA, Getty CJ. Acute compartment syndrome following revisional arthroplasty of the forefoot: the dangers of ankle-block. Foot Ankle Int 2000; 21(8):680–2.

18. Mendelson S, Mendelson A, Holmes J. Compartment syndrome after acute rupture of the peroneus longus in a high school football player: a case report. Am J Orthop 2003;32(10):510–2.

19. Andermahr J, Helling HJ, Rehm KE, et al. The vascularization of the os calcaneum and the clinical consequences. Clin Orthop 1999;363:212–8.

20. Manoli A 2nd, Weber TG. Fasciotomy of the foot: an anatomical study with special reference to release of the calcaneal compartment. Foot Ankle 1990;10(5):267–75.

21. Perry MD, Manoli A 2nd. Foot compartment syndrome. Orthop Clin North Am 2001;32(1):103–11.

22. Shereff MJ. Compartment syndromes of the foot. Instr Course Lect 1990;39:127–32.

23. Manoli A 2nd. Compartment syndromes of the foot: current concepts. Foot Ankle 1990;10(6):340–4.

24. Fulkerson E, Razi A, Tejwani N. Review: acute compartment syndrome of the foot. Foot Ankle Int 2003;24(2):180–7.

25. Karlstrom G, Lonnerholm T, Olerud S. Cavus deformity of the foot after fracture of the tibial shaft. J Bone Joint Surg Am 1975;57(7):893–900.

26. Manoli A 2nd, Fakhouri AJ, Weber TG. Concurrent compartment syndromes of the foot and leg. Foot Ankle 1993;14(6):339–42.

27. Viau MR, Pedersen HE, Salcicioli GG, et al. Ectopic calcification as a late sequela of compartment syndrome: report of two cases. Clin Orthop 1983;176:178–80.

28. Matsen FA III, Clawson DK. The deep posterior compartmental syndrome of the leg. J Bone Joint Surg Am 1975;57(1):34–9.

29. Manoli A. What happens if you do nothing? Presented at the AOFAS 21st Annual Summer Meeting. Boston, July 15–17, 2005.
30. Younger AS Hansen ST Jr, Adult cavovarus foot. J Am Acad Orthop Surg 2005;13(5): 302–15.
31. Clawson DK. Claw toes following tibial fracture. Clin Orthop 1974;103:47–8.
32. Jose RM, Viswanathan N, Aldlyami E, et al. A spontaneous compartment syndrome in a patient with diabetes. J Bone Joint Surg Br 2004;86(7):1068–70.

Postoperative Infections:
Prevention and Management

R. Glenn Gaston, MD[a,b,]*, Marshall A. Kuremsky, MD[c]

KEYWORDS

- Postoperative • Infection • Hand • Osteomyelitis • Wrist

KEY POINTS

- Postoperative infections continue to be a challenging Problem, and the incidence of bacterial antibiotic resistance such as MRSA is rising.
- There are numerous intrinsic patient factors that should be optimized before surgery to minimize the risk of SSIs.
- When postoperative infections develop, treatment must be individualized; however, the principles outlined in this article can help guide treatment.

More than 290,000 surgical site infections (SSIs) are reported annually in the United States according to recent reports from the Centers for Disease Control and Prevention (CDC). Annual direct and indirect cost estimates as a result of SSIs are in excess of $1 billion and $10 billion, respectively. An SSI has been defined by the CDC as an infection occurring within 30 days of an operative procedure or within 1 year in the event of material implantation.[1,2] These infections can be further classified as either superficial (confined to the skin and subcutaneous tissues around the incision) or deep (involving the fascia, muscle, bone, or implant). The most common causative organism involved with SSIs parallels that found in normal skin flora and is *Staphylococcus aureus*. A recent epidemiologic study[3] reported that in adults, 50% to 80% of SSI isolates are pure *S aureus*, with 12% mixed flora. Gram-negative organisms are more common in immunocompromised hosts such as people with diabetes and intravenous drug abusers.

Recently there has been an alarming and increasing trend toward methicillin-resistant *S aureus* (MRSA) isolates in SSIs. In a review of 761 patients in a 3-year period from 2001 to 2003,[4] the incidence of community-acquired MRSA in hand

A version of this article was previously published in *Hand Clinics* 26:4.

The authors have no financial disclosures or funding related to this manuscript to report.

[a] Carolinas Medical Center, 1000 Blythe Boulevard Charlotte, NC 28203, USA; [b] OrthoCarolina, 1915 Randolph Road, Charlotte, NC 28207, USA; [c] Department of Orthopedics, Carolinas Medical Center, Charlotte, NC 28203, USA

* Corresponding author. OrthoCarolina, 1915 Randolph Road, Charlotte, NC 28207.

E-mail address: glenngaston@hotmail.com

doi:10.1016/j.ccell.2012.03.007

infections nearly doubled from 34% to 61%. The incidence of MRSA has risen so dramatically that some investigators have implied that all patients presenting with hand infections should be empirically treated for MRSA.[5]

The hand is resistant to the development of infection compared with the rest of the human body; however, its uniquely intricate and confined anatomy renders it prone to significant impairment as a result of even seemingly trivial infections. SSI rates in elective hand surgery are reported to be less than 1.4%, with deep infections less than 0.3%.[6] Unlike other infections elsewhere in the body, hand infections occur frequently in the absence of fever or increased laboratory markers of infection. A recent study found that more than 75% of patients with active hand infections were afebrile and without increased C-reactive protein (CRP) and only 50% had an increased erythrocyte sedimentation rate (ESR).[3] Clinical examination therefore is of paramount importance in the diagnosis of hand infections. Delays in treatment of hand infections in particular can have devastating consequences because of the proximity of nearby critical anatomic structures to which local infection can easily spread. Dense vascular and lymph anastomoses, tendon sheaths, and deep palmar spaces all provide easy access for rapid spread of infection.

To minimize the morbidity of SSIs one must focus on modification of preoperative, intraoperative, and postoperative risk factors. If despite these efforts an SSI occurs, prompt diagnosis and management are critical. This article focuses first on the prevention of SSI through modifiable preoperative, intraoperative, and postoperative factors and second on managing established postoperative infections.

PREOPERATIVE MODIFIABLE RISK FACTORS

Numerous modifiable preoperative risk factors have been identified and associated with increased infection risk.[7–9] These risk factors include malnutrition, smoking, anemia, MRSA carrier status, obesity, poor oral health, remote infection, and systemic diseases such as diabetes, human immunodeficiency virus (HIV), and rheumatoid arthritis (RA). In an elective surgical setting, many of these risk factors can be identified and optimized before surgery.

MALNUTRITION

Malnutrition is a well-recognized risk factor for deep infections in orthopedic surgery. Typically malnutrition is defined as serum albumin level less than 3.5 g/dL, total lymphocyte count less than 1500/mm^3, or a serum transferrin level less than 226 mg/dL, and wound healing complications have been associated with these levels of malnutrition. The association of malnutrition with SSI is likely multifactorial. Decreased lymphocyte counts directly decrease host cell-mediated immunity. A lack of essential vitamins and minerals such as vitamin A, vitamin C, zinc, and copper contribute indirectly toward diminished function of T lymphocytes and natural killer cells.[10,11] Furthermore, low protein levels lead to decreased angiogenesis, increased third-space fluid losses, and poor blood oxygenation.[10] In 1 study of 31 postoperative orthopedic wound complications, 27 were found to be nutritionally depleted as defined in this article.[12]

SMOKING

Smoking continues to be the leading cause of preventable morbidity and mortality in the United States. Despite the well-known risks incurred with cigarette use, there are still more than 50 million smokers consuming in excess of 800 billion cigarettes annually in the United States.[13] By virtue of its vasoconstrictive effects and tissue-induced hypoxia, smoking can also increase risk of complications with wound healing also. The tissue-induced hypoxia from smoking is caused by the binding of carbon monoxide to hemoglobin, forming carboxyhemoglobin, which deprives local tissue of available oxygen. A randomized study has shown that smoking cessation even as little as 4 to 6 weeks preoperatively can decrease postoperative complications, including with wound healing.[14]

MRSA CARRIER

S aureus is the most common organism found in SSIs, and Staphylococcus epidermidis is often associated with infections involving implants. The incidence of community-acquired MRSA in hand infections has been steadily rising in the United States.[15] The most common strain of community-acquired MRSA, termed USA 300 by the CDC, has a unique membrane toxin named Panton-Valentine leukocidin that targets host leukocytes, resulting in often severe skin infections and antibiotic resistance.[16,17]

Nasal carriage of S aureus has been associated with 2 to 9 times increased risk of SSIs.[18] Preoperative nasal swabs for Staphylococcus and specifically MRSA have recently been developed with decolonization protocols consisting of mupirocin or Bactroban ointment applied twice daily to the nares. The authors have begun using this preoperative screening protocol on all patients with major arthroplasty, including elbow and wrist arthroplasty. If swabs are positive, vancomycin is our preoperative antibiotic of choice on the day of surgery.

DIABETES

Given population prevalence estimates of nearly 10% in the United States in adults more than 50 years old, diabetes mellitus warrants special consideration.[19] Between 5% and 35% of patients requiring hospital admission for hand infections have diabetes.[20–23] A study by Mandell[24] found that 8 of 15 presumed nondiabetic patients who had recently resolved hand infections tested positive to a glucose tolerance test, suggesting a potentially high incidence of undiagnosed diabetes in this patient population.

Diabetes has been shown to affect host cell-mediated immunity, neutrophil and lymphocyte function, and wound healing.[25] However, high levels of hyperglycemia (>250 mg/dL) and metabolic acidosis are required to produce these cellular changes.[26,27] Many potentially confounding variables such as patient age, obesity, malnutrition, local tissue hypoxia caused by poor circulation, and peripheral neuropathy likely contribute also to the high association of diabetic patients with wound healing complications, including SSI. Some studies have attempted to eliminate these confounding variables using multivariate regression analysis and have found diabetes is not an independent risk factor for the development of an SSI.[28,29] Other studies have documented higher rates of SSI in patients with diabetes even after only minor soft-tissue procedures.[30,31] Evidence is now emerging from the cardiothoracic literature that tight perioperative glycemic control directly leads to a decreased incidence of SSI and mortality.[32–34]

Patients with diabetes mellitus are not only potentially more prone to developing infections but also have a higher morbidity and mortality associated with the development of infection. In the presence of an upper-extremity infection, patients with diabetes can have amputation rates up to 63% and a mortality of 19%.[35,36] In the subset of patients with diabetes with renal failure, even higher morbidity and mortality exist, with 1 study reporting an amputation rate of 100% in this cohort.[36] In the setting of infection in a patient with diabetes, early and aggressive treatment is necessary as the severity and extent of infection are frequently underestimated in this patient population.[23] Incisions should extend along the entire length of indurated or erythematous skin.

Although S aureus remains the most common offending pathogen, fungal, polymicrobial, and gram-negative organisms (73% in some studies) have a higher prevalence in patients with diabetes.[37] Cultures for atypical mycobacterium, fungal, and anaerobic organisms are recommended in diabetic infection, and empiric antibiotic therapy needs to be broad-spectrum.

During the perioperative period, attempts to maintain serum glucose levels between 100 and 180 mg/dL should be made to optimize the immune status and wound healing potential of patients with diabetes.

HIV

HIV suppresses the formation of CD4 T-helper cells that control cell-mediated immunity. Progressive decline in CD4 cells directly correlates with the severity of the immunocompromised state and susceptibility to infection. Much like patients with diabetes, HIV-positive patients have higher morbidity associated with infections, especially in the presence of AIDS. Although the clinical presentation is similar to non-HIV-positive patients, the course of the infection tends to be unusually aggressive. Glickel[38] termed this finding as "atypical manifestations of infection with typical organisms." In Glickel's series, 7 of 8 patients had opportunistic infections elsewhere (predominantly pneumonia), whereas none had opportunistic infections of the hand.

This aggressive nature of hand infections in HIV-positive patients becomes evident considering the reoperation rate for infection has been reported to be 29% and amputation rate 12%.[39] The high rate of intravenous drug abuse in patients with HIV is an independent risk factor for the development of infection, particularly more severe or atypical infections. Herpetic viral infections are also more common in HIV-positive patients and are more virulent in this population, with a predilection for superinfection. Necrotizing fasciitis is more frequent in this population also, with an incidence of more than 20% in 1 recent study, although intravenous drug abuse is a confounding variable. Wound healing has not been found to be impaired in patients with HIV.[40,41] Hand surgeons should be cognizant also that in more than half of the reported cases, hand infection preceded the diagnosis of HIV in 1 series; therefore a high index of suspicion is necessary in such circumstances.[38]

RA

RA is an inflammatory arthropathy that affects 1% of the population.[42] There is a predilection for hand and upper-extremity involvement in RA, and SSI has a well-known association with RA surgery. In the literature for hip and knee arthroplasty, a two- to threefold increased risk of an SSI and 5 times higher rates of wound dehiscence have been reported for patients with RA compared with patients with osteoarthritis.[43] Similarly, elbow arthroplasty SSI rates are higher in patients with RA, with an incidence of 7% to 9%.[44,45] The increased rate of SSI in patients with RA has been believed to be due in part to the immunosuppressive effects of the disease, the immunosuppressive effects of the medications used to treat the disease, patient malnutrition, and other comorbidities.

Medications often used in the management of RA that have been implicated as possible causes of SSI include steroids, methotrexate, and tumor necrosis factor α (TNF-α) antagonists. Steroids, such as prednisone, are commonly used in the management of RA and suppress antibody formation and phagocyte function, thereby increasing susceptibility to infection.[46] Chronic steroid administration in animal models has caused delays in skin and bone healing.[47,48] Clinical studies looking at the association of long-term steroid use and wound healing complications have conflicting reports, with some studies finding an association[49,50] and others finding no association.[51,52]

Methotrexate usage during the perioperative period has been the source of much debate.[53] Concern stems from its immunosuppressive effects and impairment in wound healing in animal studies.[54,55] In addition, some clinical studies support methotrexate cessation before surgery.[56,57] Other clinical studies have found no increased risk of complications with wound healing or SSI in patients continuing methotrexate therapy throughout the perioperative period and a decreased incidence of disease flare-ups.[49,51,52,58]

Only 2 studies have looked specifically at SSI and wound healing complications in patients with RA undergoing hand surgery on methotrexate or steroids and neither found an increased rate of complications associated with continued use of these medications throughout the perioperative period.[52,58]

A newer class of medication, TNF-α inhibitors, has recently been gaining popularity in the management of autoimmune disorders, including RA. TNF-α antagonists block the cytokine-mediated inflammatory cascade that is overexpressed in RA patients. Presently there are 3 approved TNF-α antagonists on the market: etanercept (Enbrel), infliximib (Remicade), and adalimumab (Humira). All 3 of these medications have shown superior efficacy to that of methotrexate in preventing the bone and cartilage destruction of RA.[59] Although no specific studies have investigated hand or upper-extremity infections in patients on these medications, serious infections have been seen in up to 18% of patients with RA who are receiving TNF-αtherapy.[60]

Comorbidities such as malnutrition have also been implicated in the increased prevalence of SSI and poor wound healing in patients with RA. Rayan and colleagues[61] found that malnutrition coexisted with RA in up to 75% of patients, based on serum albumin level, total lymphocyte count, triceps skin fold measurement, and midarm muscle circumference.

MASTECTOMY

Patients having previously undergone ipsilateral mastectomy with lymph node dissection were traditionally believed to have increased risk of developing an SSI as a result of localized immune impairment[62,63]; however, there is a growing body of evidence to the contrary. Hershko and Stahl[64] recently reviewed 25 cases of elective hand surgery in patients with a history of ipsilateral mastectomy with axillary lymph node dissection and found no infections or new cases of lymphedema. Similarly, 2 separate studies investigating carpal tunnel release in this patient population found no infections in a combined total of 67 cases.[65,66] Based on the available studies, this subset of patients does not seem to be at increased risk of developing an SSI; however, given the gravity of an infection in such a limb, early and aggressive treatment of any suspected cellulitis is justified.

PROPHYLACTIC ANTIBIOTICS

Many prospective, randomized trials have reported reduced rates of SSI with the use of preoperative antibiotics in patients undergoing surgery for long-bone trauma, hip fractures, and total joint arthroplasty.[67-69] In these patients a first-generation cephalosporin such as cefazolin is the antibiotic of choice in the absence of documented β-lactam allergy or known MRSA carrier status, in which case vancomycin is recommended. For cases in which β-lactam allergy is in question, skin testing for penicillin allergy is available.[70] Optimal timing of antibiotic administration is within 60 minutes of incision to ensure adequate tissue levels are present at the commencement of surgery. Studies looking at cefazolin concentration in bone at the time of incision have found levels more than 60 times the minimal inhibitory concentration.[71]

No benefit has been shown in continuing prophylactic antibiotics beyond 24 hours postoperatively in preventing SSI, and it may propagate antimicrobial resistance.[72,73]

Unlike the general orthopedic literature, the role of prophylactic antibiotics in elective hand surgery is less clear, due in part to the overall extremely low infection rate of elective hand procedures. In a report of 2337 elective upper-extremity cases Kleinert and coleagues[6] found a deep infection rate of only 0.3%. Similarly, in a report of 3620 elective carpal tunnel releases, of which 80% were performed without antibiotic administration, Hanssen and colleagues[74] found an infection rate of 0.47%. A recent prospective, randomized, double-blind, placebo-controlled study by Whittaker and colleagues[75] found no difference in the rate of infection in clean, incised hand injuries with or without the use of preoperative antibiotics.

The literature does, however, have some evidence supporting the use of prophylactic antibiotics in specific elective hand procedures based on the length of procedure, specific host factors, presence of certain implants, and degree of wound contamination.[76] Procedures lasting more than 2 hours have been shown to have significantly increased risk of developing an SSI. Haley and colleagues[77] reviewed more than 58,000 surgical cases and found operative time of more than 2 hours to be an independent predictor of wound infection. Two additional studies provide level 1 evidence supporting the use of preoperative antibiotics in elective cases lasting more than 2 hours to minimize the risk of SSI.[78,79] It is therefore recommended that prophylactic antibiotics be given in all cases estimated to be of longer than 2 hours' duration.

The authors have recently synthesized all of the pertinent literature on antibiotic use for elective hand procedures and developed an algorithm through the quality-improvement program at our institution, which we are presently implementing. This algorithm is presented in **Fig. 1** and contains the references for the rationale for each step in the algorithm.

INTRAOPERATIVE MODIFIABLE RISK FACTORS

Intraoperative factors play an important role in the prevention of SSIs. Two recent review articles, by Fletcher and colleagues[90] and Evans,[91] detail these factors and should be referred to for more in-depth review. This summary highlights skin preparation, hair removal, wound irrigation, and postoperative drains in particular, as these issues play prominent roles in the prevention of postoperative infections within hand surgery.

PREOPERATIVE SKIN PREPARATION

Clear evidence exists supporting the use of topical skin antiseptic agents before surgical procedures.[91] Although many products are available, the most commonly used substances contain 1 of 3 primary components: iodophors (eg, povidone-iodine), chlorhexidine gluconate, or alcohol.[90,92] In clean surgery, as is frequently the case for elective procedures of the hand, a Cochrane Database review[93] showed no difference among the various skin antiseptics.

The mechanism of action for each of these agents differs.[27] The iodophors have activity against routine skin flora. Their efficacy is enhanced by permitting oxidation in room air for a few minutes after application. Their duration of activity is shorter compared with chlorhexidine gluconate.[94] Blood and related products may impart some level of inactivity on these compounds.

Chlorhexidine gluconate has been shown to have a longer duration of activity against typical skin flora compared with the iodophors.[90] It destroys bacterial cell membranes and remains active in the presence of blood proteins. It has a long duration of activity and its efficacy continues after application.[95]

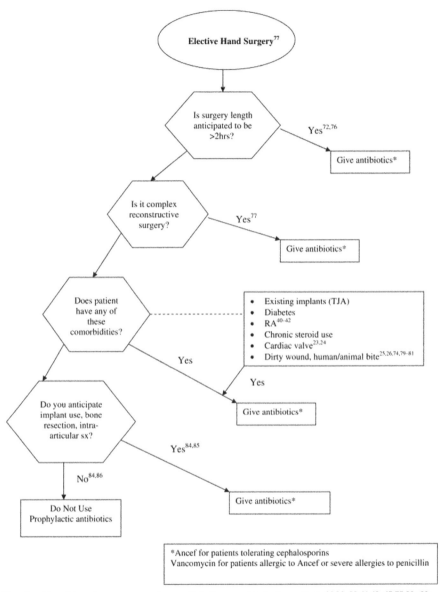

Fig. 1. Algorithm for preoperative antibiotic use. (*Data from* Refs.[14,26–29,41,43–45,75,80–89])

Alcohol has activity against bacteria, viruses, and fungi. There are concerns related to the flammability of this substance as it pertains to patient and surgeon safety. It has a relative lack of residual activity also, which may be relevant in procedures of longer duration. There is a 95% immediate reduction in skin flora on application; this can be increased to 99% if the applications are repeated.[96]

In a quantitative assessment of skin contamination on feet, Keblish and colleagues[97] found that use of a brush, compared with a standard applicator, was more efficacious in reducing positive cultures from web spaces. This finding may have applicability to the hand, particularly in nonelective or trauma procedures in which there may be more inherent debris or contamination on the skin at the time of preparation.

PREOPERATIVE HAIR REMOVAL

Although removal of hair at the surgical site before the procedure is a common practice, there remains a paucity of evidence to support its use.[90] The proposed benefit of hair removal includes shortening the hair (such that the length available for bacterial colonization and contamination is diminished) and removing hair from an area of a planned incision that may create additional debris in the surgical site or may be entrapped in the incision during wound closure. Shaving on the night before the operation is not recommended because of an increased risk of SSI secondary to microscopic lesions in the epidermis, which can then retain bacteria.[98] Razor use more than 24 hours before surgery has been associated with an infection risk of 20%.[99] When the hair is to be cut before surgery clippers are preferred to use of a razor. Clippers do not come into contact with the skin, and some studies have associated their use with a decrease in postoperative infection rates.[91,100–102]

Preoperative hair removal has been studied in a meta-analysis by the Cochrane group.[103] There was a significantly higher relative risk (nearly double) of SSI following hair removal with a razor compared with clippers. These data revealed no difference in infection rate whether hair was removed before a procedure or not, suggesting that refraining from hair removal before surgery does not necessarily predispose to increase risk of SSI. In a study by Seropian and Reynolds,[104] the lowest SSI rates (0.6%) were noted with use of a depilatory agent or with no hair removal at all. As an alternative, depilatory products may also be used in lieu of clippers; these products can remove a significant amount of hair without creating microabrasions in the skin that may increase risk for infection.

WOUND IRRIGATION

The use of intraoperative wound irrigation in clean surgery is another technique that may minimize SSIs.[90] In a study of patients undergoing spine surgery, there is a significant difference in the infection rate in patients who underwent wound irrigation with a povidone-iodine (0.5% infection rate) irrigant compared with those who did not (2.9%).[105] The addition of antibiotics to the irrigant solution has been common historically, although this practice is not clearly justified in the literature.[106] Significant debate continues as to whether pulsatile lavage versus bulb syringe has greater efficacy, particularly in dirty or contaminated wounds.[91] Pulsatile lavage may offer benefits in being able to deliver higher-pressure irrigation, which may be useful when debris are impacted into the soft tissue or are not grossly apparent during debridement; alternatively some investigators believe that high-pressure lavage may cause deeper penetration of bacteria within tissues, preventing its removal.[107] High-pressure pulsatile lavage may also damage bone, and thus theoretically impair healing also.[91] Other investigators have shown that high-pressure lavage can result in deep seeding of the bone or medullary canal itself.[108,109]

There is some evidence for the use of detergents, such as castile soap or benzalkonium chloride, in wound irrigation fluid. The unique feature of detergents is their ability to disrupt the forces (electrostatic and hydrophobic) that otherwise bind bacteria to human tissue.[91] In a prospective, randomized study by Anglen,[110] more than 400 open fractures of the lower extremity were irrigated with either bacitracin or castile soap. In this study, there was no difference in rates of SSI or bone healing between the 2 groups, but there was more than a twofold difference in rate of wound healing for those open fractures irrigated with bacitracin compared with castile soap.

DRAINS

Wound closure over a drain has not been proven to lower SSI rates.[90,91] Much of the literature investigating this topic has been performed in joint arthroplasty. In a study by Beer and colleagues,[111] no difference in drainage, infection, or swelling was noted in patients with bilateral knee arthroplasties with and without drains. Furthermore, a meta-analysis by Parker and colleagues[112] of more than 3600 arthroplasty wounds showed no major benefit to use of a drain in hip or knee replacement surgery, but did show a higher need for transfusion with use of a drain.

Closed suction drains are associated with less retrograde bacterial migration compared with simple conduit drains.[113] Studies have shown that wound infections are associated with contaminated drain tips; however, negative culture of drain tips is not commonly associated with surgical wound infection.[114] There does seem to be a time-dependent phenomenon associated with duration of indwelling drains and wound infection; multiple studies have shown that drains left in wounds for more than 24 hours have a higher association with wound infections.[115,116]

MANAGEMENT OF SSIs

Despite all our efforts to prevent SSI, postoperative infections will continue to occur. Although there are important general principles to follow in dealing with SSI, the treatment plan must be individualized. The first step in the management of a potential SSI is to obtain a thorough history and physical examination. The timeline for onset of symptoms should be ascertained, as earlier detection has a higher likelihood of successful management with proper immobilization and oral antibiotics alone. Also, the rapidity of symptom progression is critical, especially when considering aggressive rapidly progressing infections such as necrotizing fasciitis. The presence of hardware and stability of the underlying fracture when present must be considered. The host risk factors outlined earlier must be considered and included in the decision for potentially more aggressive management. In posttraumatic cases, the nature of the injury, especially as it relates to possible sources of infection, must be sought (eg, bite wound, soil contamination, marine environment) to help guide empiric antibiotic selection.

Physical examination should focus first on differentiating a superficial from a deep infection. The most common superficial infection is cellulitis, which manifests as erythema, warmth, swelling, tenderness, and at times loss of motion. Cellulitis can progress along lymphatic tracks, causing an ascending lymphangitis, which appears as red streaking up the arm. Regional lymphadenopathy and tenderness should be assessed about the medial epicondyle and axilla. Particular attention should be paid to assess for any areas of fluctuance, induration, or subcutaneous crepitation to suggest an underlying abscess or fasciitis, which would require prompt surgical decompression. Minor cellulitis can most often be managed with oral antibiotics such as Keflex or clindamycin (for penicillin allergy) to provide coverage for the 2 most common organisms, *Streptococcus* and *Staphylococcus*. For suspected MRSA, the only currently approved oral antibiotic by the Food and Drug Administration is linezolid; however, several studies have reported success with trimethoprim-sulfamethoxazole (Bactrim). Linezolid (Zyvox) is a new class of antibiotic known as oxazolidinone, designed specifically for MRSA and vancomycin-resistant *Enterococcus faecium*. It has been shown to have excellent penetration of bone and soft tissue, with nearly 100% bioavailability by mouth. Despite these excellent antimicrobial properties, the authors reserve the use of Zyvox for only the most extreme cases because of its high cost. When considering oral treatment for suspected or culture-positive MRSA, we typically favor Bactrim DS (2 tablets twice daily).

In postoperative infection suspected to be confined to the subcutaneous tissue, initial management with immobilization, elevation, and antibiotics is appropriate. Progress should be monitored closely and if improvement is not seen in 24 to 48 hours the patient should be reassessed for possible deep-space infection or the need for intravenous antibiotics.

Advanced imaging studies in the acute postoperative infection are rarely necessary, but in more indolent presentations can be useful. Advanced imaging can also be of benefit in distinguishing superficial infections from deeper infections when the physical diagnosis is in question. Ultrasound can help identify deeper fluid collections and guide aspiration. MRI can be of great benefit, particularly in the absence of metallic hardware, in determining deep tissue involvement such as deep abscess or osteomyelitis.

If deep infection is suspected on examination or by imaging studies, surgical drainage is necessary. Cultures should be obtained at the time of debridement and antibiotic therapy tailored to the organism and extent of infection present. Antibiotic therapy should be delayed until after cultures are obtained if possible to improve culture sensitivity. If suspicion is high for an atypical organism (eg, marine environment, immunocompromised host) special media and agar plating may be necessary and the laboratory should be alerted in advance of culture delivery to increase likelihood of culture-positive results.

When surgical drainage is deemed to be necessary, careful planning of incisions is needed to avoid possible exposed hardware, tendons, or nerves. Often this is dictated by the original incision in the acute postoperative period following an open procedure, but for percutaneous surgeries or more remote SSIs more latitude exists. When possible in the digits the authors prefer midlateral incisions along the nonborder surface of the finger. In keeping with general orthopedic principles, a thorough debridement is necessary of all nonviable tissue. Wounds are then typically left open to heal by secondary intention or only loosely closed over vital structures, with drains kept in place. For larger open wounds in the hand and forearm the wound vacuum-assisted closure (VAC, Kinetic Concept Inc, San Antonio, TX, USA) has proved useful.[117]

WOUND VAC

In situations in which primary wound closure is either not possible or not desired (in favor of delayed primary closure or healing by secondary intention), the authors have found the VAC an invaluable resource. The VAC is contraindicated in the presence of untreated osteomyelitis or malignancy. The concept of the VAC was first introduced in 1997 and involves the placement of a reticulated polyurethane sponge covered with an airtight occlusive dressing and connected to a suction canister by tubing.[118] Negative pressure can then be applied. The dressing is typically changed every 2 to 3 days at the bedside unless additional operative debridement is necessary.

When applied in the setting of an SSI, the principles of thorough wound debridement must be adhered to before VAC application. Once the wound has been meticulously debrided, vital structures such as nerves and tendons should be covered with local tissue or muscle to avoid desiccation and vessels covered with local tissue or muscle to avoid hemorrhage. Catastrophic hemorrhage has been reported when the VAC was applied in contact with vessels.[119]

The negative pressure exerted on the wound has been shown to remove edema and hemorrhage, improve local circulation, and enhance granulation tissue formation. Animal studies using laser Doppler have confirmed improved local circulation by decreasing capillary afterload.[118,120–122] This improved local perfusion leads directly to improved formation of granulation tissue. Studies comparing the VAC with traditional wet-to-dry dressings have found an 80% improvement in formation of granulation tissue.[123] Despite the theory that the VAC could remove accumulating purulence, studies have failed to report reduced bacterial loads but have reported improved wound healing from significant decreases in wound surface area.[122,124] The cost of VAC therapy is nearly identical to wet-to-dry dressings when accounting for nursing personnel dressing changes ($103 per day for VAC vs $100 per day for wet-to-dry dressings).[125]

Three specific postoperative infections deserve special consideration because of the high morbidity associated with their development and will be addressed individually: septic arthritis, osteomyelitis, and necrotizing fasciitis.

SEPTIC ARTHRITIS

Septic arthritis of the hand and wrist typically results from direct inoculation but may also arise from bactericidal or adjacent spread of a deep-space infection. Although it has received little attention in the literature, this can be a vexing complication for the patient and surgeon. Classically patients with septic arthritis present with painful swelling of the involved joint, loss of motion, and significant pain with passive motion. The joint classically postures to maximize capsular distension, which in the fingers is in a slightly flexed position. Because standard laboratory markers of infection are of less value in determining the presence of infection in the hand, aspiration should be obtained if clinical suspicion is present. Aspirate should be sent for glucose level, cell count, Gram stain, and culture to look for septic arthritis and crystal analysis to rule out gout. Septic arthritis should be suspected in cases of white blood cell (WBC) count greater than 50,000 with greater than 75% polymorphonuclear lymphocytes and a glucose concentration of 40 mg less than fasting glucose level.[126,127]

Management of septic arthritis is typically prompt surgical debridement of the involved joint to prevent articular cartilage degeneration, as outcomes have been closely tied to timing of intervention.[126] Patients presenting at more than 10 days have been shown to have universally poor results.[128] Articular cartilage degeneration and even bony erosions can occur if treatment is delayed because of continued joint exudate build-up, causing rising intra-articular pressure, which impedes synovial blood supply. Furthermore, bacterial toxins and proteolytic enzymes directly degrade articular cartilage.[126]

If patients present early (<24 hours from symptom onset), initial management with intravenous antibiotics, immobilization, and elevation is appropriate with close observation. Empiric antibiotics should again target *Staphylococcus* and *Streptococcus* species, as these are the most common pathogens. In the event of symptom progression or lack of significant improvement over the first 24 to 48 hours the patient should undergo operative exploration and drainage. Should surgery be necessary, preoperative planning of incisions to avoid resultant exposed joint, tendons, or neurovascular structures is critical.

In the wrist, a midline dorsal incision is used followed by arthrotomy between the third and fourth compartments. A recent trend toward arthroscopic debridement of septic arthritis of the wrist has developed, with results reported superior to open techniques with respect to length of hospital stay and need for repeat surgeries.[129]

For the metacarpophalangeal joints of the hand, the authors prefer a dorsal incision and then accessing the joint with an extensor splitting approach although often a traumatic arthrotomy is present through which the joint can be accessed. Release of the proximal aspect of the sagittal band fibers is also an appropriate method.

For the interphalangeal joints of the hand, we prefer a midlateral approach to access the joint either between the extensor mechanism and proper collateral ligament or between the accessory collateral ligament and volar plate. Avoiding the extensor mechanism at this level can help minimize the risk of iatrogenic swan neck or boutonniere deformity. Care must be taken, however, to avoid injury to the neurovascular bundle, which can be displaced as a result of significant digital swelling.

The skin is always left open to heal by secondary intention or closed loosely over a drain with the hand and wrist splinted in a position of function and elevated. Intravenous antibiotics are continued until systemic and local signs of infection have resolved, then a transition to oral antibiotics based on culture results for an additional 2 to 4 weeks is warranted.[127] Early hand therapy (preferably within 2 days) should be instituted as loss of motion is a significant problem, especially in the early postoperative period.[130]

OSTEOMYELITIS

By definition osteomyelitis is an infection involving bone. Osteomyelitis of the hand and wrist is rare compared with other locations in the body, accounting for less than 10% of reported cases. Postoperative osteomyelitis has been reported in 0% to 2.5% of hand cases following internal fixation of fractures.[131,132] Osteomyelitis can also result from direct extension of septic arthritis or deep abscess into bone and in rare cases by hematogenous spread or pin-track infection. Again *Staphylococcus* and *Streptococcus* are the most common organisms.

Presentation can be more subtle than other hand infections but include local erythema, swelling, warmth, tenderness, loss of motion, and at times a draining sinus. Systemic symptoms are rare. Although most patients will have local signs of inflammation, it has been reported that only one-third may have fever or increased WBC counts.[133] In cases of acute osteomyelitis, radiographs are typically negative, with the earliest radiographic sign being swelling of the soft tissue. Two or 3 weeks later, osteopenia, sclerosis, and periosteal reactions may be seen. In chronic cases, sequestrum (focus of necrotic bone) and involucrum may be seen. Many advanced imaging modalities have been used to diagnose osteomyelitis. Overall, the sensitivity and specificity of these tests is lower than might be expected for peripheral, chronic cases of osteomyelitis (**Table 1**).[134] Bone biopsy and culture remain the gold standard for diagnosis.

Although in some cases acute osteomyelitis may be effectively managed with antibiotics alone before sequestrum formation, most cases are best managed with a combined surgical and medical treatment. Surgery should be approached similar to a tumor case with an emphasis on adequate thorough debridement of all nonviable tissue. A salvage protocol must then encompass systemic or local antibiotics, skeletal stability, soft-tissue coverage, and bone grafting.[135] A complete review of this reconstructive ladder is beyond the scope of this article but a review by Zalavras and colleagues[135] should be referred to. In cases of retained hardware, stability of the bone and hardware must be assessed. If the fracture is healed and stable, the hardware should be removed. If the implant is loose, it should be removed and

Table 1 Sensitivity and specificity of osteomyelitis tests		
Test	Sensitivity (%)	Specificity (%)
Positron emission tomography scan	96	91
Bone scan	82	25
Labeled WBC scan	84	80
Magnetic resonance imaging	84	60

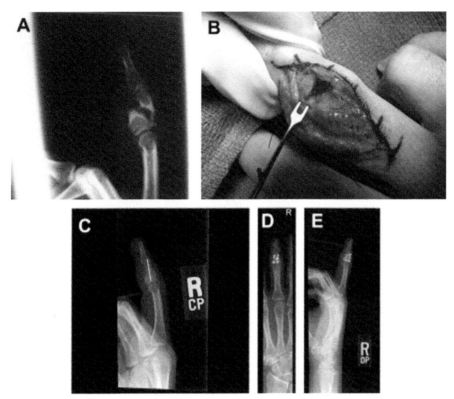

Fig. 2. (*A*) Preoperative lateral radiograph of middle phalanx osteomyelitis. (*B*) Intraoperative photograph following debridement. (*C*) Postoperative lateral with antibiotic polymethylmethacrylate (PMMA) spacer in place. (*D*) Final anteroposterior radiograph after removal of spacer and iliac crest graft placement. (*E*) Final lateral radiograph.

external fixation applied if the bone is unstable. If hardware is well fixed, an individualized approach must be used with either hardware retention with suppressive antibiotics until fracture union or hardware removal, external fixation, and possible late hardware replacement. When possible, hardware removal is favored because of the protective barrier known as biofilm associated with implants that renders antibiotic therapy less effective.

In patients in whom segments of bone require removal, cement spacers impregnated with an antibiotic can be a useful adjunct to maintain bone and soft-tissue length and provide local antibiotic delivery. Late reconstruction is then planned based on the size of the structural defect, with most cases involving less than 6-cm defects being amenable to autogenous iliac crest bone grafts and cases greater than 6 cm often necessitating vascularized grafts such as free fibula transfer (**Figs. 2** and **3**).

Prolonged intravenous antibiotics are frequently required for a 4- to 6-week minimum based on the severity of the infection and virulence of the organism. ESR and CRP levels can be helpful to follow eradication of infection. Despite aggressive management, osteomyelitis (especially of the tubular bones of the hand) can lead to marked disability, with amputation rates approaching 40% in some studies.[136]

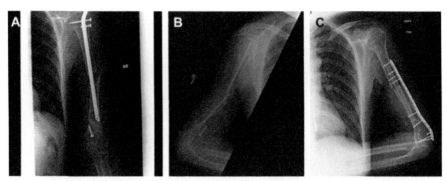

Fig. 3. (*A*) Humeral shaft osteomyelitis following intramedullary rod placement. (*B*) Postdebridement and placement of antibiotic PMMA spacer with intramedullary component. (*C*) Final radiograph following free fibula reconstruction.

NECROTIZING FASCIITIS

Necrotizing fasciitis is a rapidly advancing life-threatening infection of the skin, subcutaneous tissue, and fascia. There is a predilection for involvement of the extremities and a high association with intravenous drug use (63% in 1 study).[137] Based on the bacteriology, 2 types of necrotizing fasciitis have been described. Type 1 infection is most common (80% of cases) and is caused by mixed aerobic and anaerobic bacteria, including nongroup A streptococci. Type 2 infections are caused by group A streptococci alone or in combination with *Staphylococcus* species.[138]

Initially, necrotizing fasciitis may present similar to cellulitis with erythema and swelling but typically with more intense focal pain. Pain with palpation outside the zone of cellulitis should heighten concern for possible necrotizing fasciitis. Often more extensive nonpitting edema is present beyond the zone of erythema with tense, shiny skin. As the infection spreads, the initial zone of involvement grows, assumes a darker dusky hue (often gray in appearance), bullae may begin to appear, the skin may become anesthetic, subcutaneous crepitation may rarely be palpable, complaints of pain intensify, and hemodynamic instability may ensue **Fig. 4**.[139] These infections can spread rapidly, even in a few hours, and early adequate surgical debridement is the cornerstone of treatment.

Surgical debridement must be extensive (typically far beyond the expected zone of involvement). Findings of a fibrinous, necrotic tissue with what has been called "dish-water pus" tracking along the fascial plane are diagnostic. Subcutaneous vessel thrombosis and liquefaction of subcutaneous fat is typically present also. Blunt finger dissection along the involved fascial planes is easily accomplished. Wide debridement of all nonviable skin, subcutaneous fat, fascia, and at times muscle is critical, with amputation sometimes necessary. Moist dressings should then be applied and wounds left open with subsequent operative debridements every 1 to 2 days until the patient and wound have stabilized and all nonviable tissue has been excised. Multiple debridements are typically necessary and coverage with skin grafts or flaps common. Intense medical management for fluid resuscitation and broad-spectrum intravenous antibiotics are needed. Despite aggressive management, mortality ranges from 33% to 76% even in healthy young adults, with the single most important determinant of mortality being early and adequate debridement.[137,140] Additional

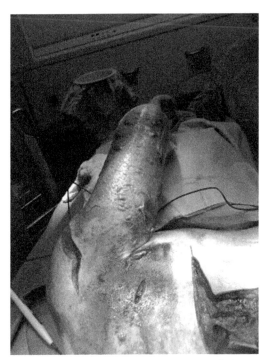

Fig. 4. Clinical photograph of necrotizing fasciitis. (*Courtesy of* Alan Ward, MD.)

negative prognostic factors of outcome include age greater than 50 years, diabetes and other chronic illnesses, and involvement of the chest wall.[140]

SUMMARY

Postoperative infections continue to be a challenging problem. The incidence of bacterial antibiotic resistance such as MRSA is rising. There are numerous intrinsic patient factors that should be optimized before surgery to minimize the risk of SSIs. When postoperative infections develop, treatment must be individualized; however, the principles outlined in this article can help guide treatment.

REFERENCES

1. Mangrum AJ, Horan TC, Pearson ML, et al. Guideline for prevention of surgical site infection, 1999. Hospital Infection Control Practices Advisory Committee. Infect Control Hosp Epidemiol 1999;20:250–78.
2. Graf K, Ott E, Vonberg RP, et al. Surgical site infections–economic consequences for the health care system. Langenbecks Arch Surg 2011;396(4):453–9.
3. Houshian S, Seyedipour S, Wedderkopp N. Epidemiology of bacterial hand infections. Int J Infect Dis 2006;10(4):315–9.
4. LeBlanc DM, Reece EM, Horton JB, et al. Increasing incidence of methicillin-resistant *Staphylococcus aureus* in hand infections: a 3-year county hospital experience. Plast Reconstr Surg 2007;119(3):935–40.
5. Wilson PC, Rinker B. The incidence of methicillin-resistant *Staphylococcus aureus* in community-acquired hand infections. Ann Plast Surg 2009;62(5):513–6.

6. Kleinert JM, Hoffman J, Miller Cran G, et al. Postoperative infection in a double-occupancy operating room. J Bone Joint Surg Am 1997;79:503–13.

7. The American Academy of Orthopedic Surgeons Patient Safety Committee, Evans RPSurgical site infection prevention and control: an emerging paradigm. J Bone Joint Surg 2009;91(6):2–9.

8. Froimson MI. Orthopedic surgical infection prevention: host and environmental factors. Am J Orthop (Belle Mead NJ) 2011;40(Suppl 12):6–9.

9. Moucha CS, Clyburn T, Evans RP, et al. Modifiable risk factors for surgical site infection. J Bone Joint Surg Am 2011;93(4):398–404.

10. Hansen P, Parvizi J. Links between malnutrition and infection are established. Orthopedics Today, November 19, 2009.

11. Fairfield KM, Fletcher RH. Vitamins for chronic disease prevention in adults: scientific review. JAMA 2002;287:3116–26.

12. Jensen JE, Jensen TG, Smith TK, et al. Nutrition in orthopaedic surgery. J Bone Joint Surg Am 1982;64(9):1263–72.

13. Porter SE, Hanley EN Jr. The musculoskeletal effects of smoking. J Am Acad Orthop Surg 2001;9(1):9–17.

14. Lindgren L. Postoperative orthopaedic infections in patients with diabetes mellitus. Acta Orthop Scand 1973;44:149–51.

15. Kiran RV, McCampbell B, Angeles AP, et al. Increased prevalence of community-acquired methicillin-resistant *Staphylococcus aureus* in hand infections at an urban medical centre. Plast Reconstr Surg 2006;118:161.

16. Lina G, Piemont Y, Godail-Gamot F, et al. Involvement of Panton-Valentine leukocidin-producing *Staphylococcus aureus* in primary skin infections and pneumonia. Clin Infect Dis 1999;29:1128–32.

17. McDougal LK, Steward CD, Killgore GE, et al. Pulsed-field gel electrophoresis typing of oxacillin-resistant *Staphylococcus* isolates from United States: establishing a national database. J Clin Microbiol 2003;41:5113–20.

18. Morange-Saussier V, Giraudeau B, Van der Mee N, et al. Nasal carriage of methicillin-resistant *Staphylococcus aureus* in vascular surgery. Ann Vasc Surg 2006;20:767–72.

19. Calvet H, Yoshikawa T. Infections in diabetes. Infect Dis Clin North Am 2001;15:407–21.

20. Stern PJ, Staneck JL, McDonough JJ, et al. Established hand infections: a controlled, prospective study. J Hand Surg 1983;8:553.

21. Glass KD. Factors related to the resolution of treated hand infections. J Hand Surg 1982;7:388

22. Maloon S, deBeer JV, Opitz M, et al. Acute flexor tendon sheath infections. J Hand Surg 1990;15:474

23. Gunther SF, Gunther SB. Diabetic hand infections. Hand Clin 1998;14(4):647–56.

24. Mandell MA. Hand infections and diabetes mellitus. Contemp Orthop 1979;1:25.

25. Phillips LG, Geldner P, Brou J. Correction of diabetic incisional healing impairment with basic fibroblast growth factor. Surg Forum 1990;41:602.

26. Shapiro DB. Postoperative infection in hand surgery: cause, prevention, and treatment. Hand Clin 1994;10:1–2.

27. Shapiro DB. Postoperative infection in hand surgery. Hand Clin 1998;14(4):669–81.

28. Culver DH, Horan TC, Gaynes RP, et al. Surgical wound infection rates by wound class, operative procedure, and patient risk index. National Nosocomial Infections Surveillance System. Am J Med 1991;91(Suppl 3B):152S–7.

29. Garibaldi RA, Cushing D, Lerer T. Risk factors for post-operative infection. Am J Med 1991;91:158S–63.

30. Gleckman R, Al-Wawi M. A review of selective infections in the adult diabetic. Compr Ther 1999;25:109–13.

31. Gonzalez MH, Bochar S, Novotny J, et al. Upper extremity infections in patients with diabetes mellitus. J Hand Surg 1999;24(4):682–6.

32. Furnary AP, Gao G, Grunkemeier GL, et al. Continuous insulin infusion reduces mortality in patients with diabetes undergoing coronary artery bypass grafting. J Thorac Cardiovasc Surg 2003;125(5):1007–21.

33. Furnary AP, Zerr KJ, Grunkemeier GL, et al. Continuous intravenous insulin infusion reduces the incidence of deep sternal wound infection in diabetic patients after cardiac surgical procedures. Ann Thorac Surg 1999;67(2):352–60.

34. Zerr KJ, Furnary AP, Grunkemeier GL, et al. Glucose control lowers the risk of wound infection in diabetics after open heart operations. Ann Thorac Surg 1997;63(2):356–61.

35. Benotmane A, Faraoun K, Mohammedi F. Infections of the upper extremity in hospitalized diabetic patients: a prospective study. Diabetes Metab 2004;30(1): 91–7.

36. Francel TJ, Marshall KA, Savage RC. Hand infections in the diabetic and the diabetic renal transplant recipient. Ann Plast Surg 1990;24(4):304–9.

37. Kour AK, Looi KP, Phone MH, et al. Hand infections in patients with diabetes. Clin Orthop Relat Res 1996;331:238–44.

38. Glickel SZ. Hand infections in patients with acquired immunodeficiency syndrome. J Hand Surg 1988;13(5):770.

39. Gonzalez MH, Nikoleit J, Weinzweig N, et al. Upper extremity infections in patients with the human immunodeficiency virus. J Hand Surg Am 1998;23:348–52.

40. Buehrer JL, Weber DJ, Meyer AA, et al. Wound infection rates after invasive procedures in HIV-1 seropositive versus HIV-1 seronegative hemophiliacs. Ann Surg 1990;211:492–8.

41. Weber DJ, Becherer PR, Rutala WA, et al. Nosocomial infection rate as a function of human immunodeficiency virus type 1 status in hemophiliacs. Am J Med 1991; 91(Suppl 3B):206S–12.

42. Akil M, Amos RS. ABC of rheumatology: rheumatoid arthritis–I: clinical features and diagnosis. BMJ 1995;310:587–90.

43. White RH, McCurdy SA, Marder RA. Early morbidity after total hip arthroplasty: rheumatoid arthritis versus osteoarthritis. J Gen Intern Med 1990;5:3034.

44. Wolfe SW, Figge MP, Ingles AE, et al. Management of infection about total elbow prosthesis. J Bone Joint Surg Am 1990;72:198–212.

45. Morrey BF, Adam R, Bryan RS. Infection after total elbow arthroplasty. J Bone Joint Surg Am 1983;65:330–8.

46. National Research Council Postoperative wound infection: the influence of ultraviolet irradiation of the operating room and various other factors. Ann Surg 1964; 160(Suppl):1–92.

47. Waters RV, Gamradt SC, Asnis P, et al. Systemic corticosteroids inhibit bone healing in a rabbit ulnar osteotomy model. Acta Orthop Scand 2000;71:316–21.

48. Cross SE, Naylor IL, Coleman RA, et al. An experimental model to investigate the dynamics of wound contraction. Br J Plast Surg 1995;48:189–97.

49. Grennan DM, Gray J, Loudon J, et al. Methotrexate and early postoperative complications in patients with rheumatoid arthritis undergoing elective orthopaedic surgery. Ann Rheum Dis 2001;60:214–7.

50. Garner RW, Mowat AG, Hazleman BL. Post-operative wound healing in patients with rheumatoid arthritis. Ann Rheum Dis 1973;32:273–4.

51. Perhala RS, Wilke WS, Clough JD, et al. Local infectious complications following large joint replacement in rheumatoid arthritis patients treated with methotrexate versus those not treated with methotrexate. Arthritis Rheum 1991;34:146–52.

52. Jain A, Witbreuk M, Ball C, et al. Influence of steroids and methotrexate on wound complications after elective hand and wrist surgery. J Hand Surg 2002;27:449–55.

53. Steuer A, Keat AC. Perioperative use of methotrexate – a survey of clinical practice in the UK. Br J Rheumatol 1997;36:1009–11.

54. Cohen SC, Gabelnick HL, Johnson RK, et al. Effects of antineoplastic agents on wound healing in mice. Surgery 1975;78:238–44.

55. Shamberger RC, Devereux DF, Brennan MF. The effect of chemotherapeutic agents on wound healing. Int Adv Surg Oncol 1981;4:15–58.

56. Bridges SL Jr, Lopez-Mendez A, Han KH, et al. Should methotrexate be discontinued before elective orthopedic surgery in patients with rheumatoid arthritis?. J Rheumatol 1991;18:984–8.

57. Carpenter MT, West SG, Vogelgesang SA, et al. Postoperative joint infections in rheumatoid arthritis patients on methotrexate therapy. Orthopedics 1996;19: 207–10.

58. Kasdan ML, June L. Postoperative results of rheumatoid arthritis patients on methotrexate at the time of reconstructive surgery of the hand. Orthopedics 1993;16: 1233–5.

59. Donahue KE, Gartlehner G, Jonas DE, et al. Systematic review: comparative effectiveness and harms of disease modifying medications for rheumatoid arthritis. Ann Intern Med 2008;148:124–34.

60. Kroesen S, Widmer AF, Tyndall A, et al. Serious bacterial infections in patients with rheumatoid arthritis under TNF-α therapy. Rheumatology 2003;42:617–21.

61. Rayan GM, McCormack ST, Hoelzer DJ, et al. Nutrition and the rheumatoid hand patient. J Okla State Med Assoc 1989;82:505.

62. Calkins ER. Nosocomial infections in hand surgery. Hand Clin 1998;14(4):531–45.

63. Simon MS, Cody RL. Cellulitis after lymph node dissection for carcinoma of the breast. Am J Med 1992;93:543.

64. Hershko DD, Stahl S. Safety of elective hand surgery following axillary lymph node dissection for breast cancer. Breast J 2007;13(3):287–90.

65. Dawson WJ, Elenz DR, Winchester DP, et al. Elective hand surgery in the breast cancer patient with prior ipsilateral axillary dissection. Ann Surg Oncol 1995;2(2): 132–7.

66. Assmus H, Staub F. [Postmastectomy lymphedema and carpal tunnel syndrome: surgical considerations and advice for patients]. Handchir Mikrochir Plast Chir 2004;36(4):237–40 [in German].

67. Boyd RJ, Burke JF, Colton T. A double-blind clinical trial of prophylactic antibiotics in hip fractures. J Bone Joint Surg Am 1973;55:1251–8.

68. Gatell JM, Riba J, Lozano ML, et al. Prophylactic cefamandole in orthopedic surgery. J Bone Joint Surg Am 1984;66:1219.

69. Schulitz KP, Winkelmann W, Schoening B. The prophylactic use of antibiotics in alloarthroplasty of the hip for coxarthrosis. Arch Orthop Trauma Surg 1980;96: 79–82.

70. Li JT, Markus PJ, Osmon DR, et al. Reduction of vancomycin use in orthopedic patients with a history of antibiotic allergy. Mayo Clin Proc 2000;75:902–6.

71. Cunha BA, Gossling HR, Pasternak HS, et al. The penetration characteristics of cefazolin, cephalothin, and cephradine into bone in patients undergoing total hip replacement. J Bone Joint Surg Am 1977;59:856–9.

72. Dellinger EP, Gross PA, Barrett TL, et al. Quality standard for antimicrobial prophylaxis in surgical procedures. Infectious Diseases Society of America. Clin Infect Dis 1994;18:422–7.

73. Oishi CS, Carrion WV, Hoaglund FT. Use of parenteral prophylactic antibiotics in clean orthopedic surgery. A review of the literature. Clin Orthop Relat Res 1972;296: 249–55.

74. Hanssen AD, Amadio PC, DeSilva SP. Deep postoperative wound infection after carpal tunnel release. J Hand Surg Am 1989;14:869–73.

75. Whittaker JP, Nancarrow JD, Sterne GD. The role of antibiotic prophylaxis in clean incised hand injuries: a prospective randomized placebo controlled double blind trial. J Hand Surg Br 2005;30:162–7.

76. Rizvi M, Bille B, Holtom P, et al. The role of prophylactic antibiotics in elective hand surgery. J Hand Surg Am 2008;33:413–20.

77. Haley RW, Culver DH, Morgan W, et al. Identifying patients at high risk of surgical wound infection. Am J Epidemiol 1985;121:206–15.

78. Classen DC, Evans RS, Pestotnik SL, et al. The timing of prophylactic administration of antibiotics and the risk of surgical wound infection. N Engl J Med 1992;326: 281–6.

79. Henley BM, Jones RE, Wyatt RWB, et al. Prophylaxis with cefamandole nafate in elective orthopedic surgery. Clin Orthop 1986;209:249–54.

80. Amland PF, Andenaes K, Smadal F, et al. A prospective, double blind, placebo controlled trial of a single dose of azithromycin on postoperative wound infections in plastic surgery. Plast Reconstr Surg 1995;96:948–56.

81. Ehrenkranz NJ. Surgical wound infection occurrence in clean operations. Am J Med 1981;70:909–14.

82. Haley RW. Nosocomial infections in surgical patients: developing valid measures of intrinsic patient risk. Am J Med 1991;91(Suppl 3B):145S–51.

83. Cummings P. Antibiotics to prevent infection in patients with dog bite wounds: a meta-analysis of randomized trials. Ann Emerg Med 1994;23:535–40.

84. Platt AJ, Page RE. Postoperative infection following hand surgery. J Hand Surg Br 1995;20:685–90.

85. Mishriki SF, Law DJW, Jeffrey PJ. Factors affecting the incidence of postoperative wound infection. J Hosp Infect 1990;16:223–30.

86. Swanson AB. Flexible implant arthroplasty for arthritic finger joints. Rationale, technique, and results of treatment. J Bone Joint Surg Am 1972;54:435–55.

87. Botte MJ, Davis JLW, Rose BA. Complications of smooth pin fixation of fractures and dislocations in the hand and wrist. Clin Orthop Relat Res 1992;276:194–201.

88. Furnes A, Havelin LI, Engesaeter LB, et al. [Quality control of prosthetic replacements of knee, ankle, toe, shoulder, elbow and finger joint in Norway 1994. A report after the first year of registration of joint prostheses in the national registry]. Tidsskr Nor Laegeforen 1996;116:177 [in Norwegian].

89. Swanson AB. Flexible implant arthroplasty in the proximal interphalangeal joint of the hand. J Hand Surg Am 1985;10:796–805.

90. Fletcher N, Sofianos D, Berkes MB, et al. Prevention of perioperative infection. J Bone Joint Surg Am 2007;89:1605–18.

91. Evans RP. Surgical site infection prevention and control: an emerging paradigm. J Bone Joint Surg Am 2009;91(Suppl 6):2–9.

92. Spillane CB, Dabo MN, Fletcher NC, et al. The dichotomy in the DNA-binding behaviour of ruthenium(II) complexes bearing benzoxazole and benzothiazole groups. J Inorg Biochem 2008;102:673–83.

93. Edwards PS, Lipp A, Holmes A. Preoperative skin antiseptics for preventing surgical wound infections after clean surgery. Cochrane Database Syst Rev 2004;3: CD003949.

94. Aly R, Maibach HI. Comparative antibacterial efficacy of a 2-minute surgical scrub with chlorhexidine gluconate, povidone-iodine, and chloroxylenol sponge-brushes. Am J Infect Control 1988;16:173–7.

95. Dahl J, Wheeler B, Mukherjee D. Effect of chlorhexidine scrub on postoperative bacterial counts. Am J Surg 1990;159:486–8.

96. Ayliffe GA. Surgical scrub and skin disinfection. Infect Control 1984;5:23–7.

97. Keblish DJ, Zurakowski D, Wilson MG, et al. Preoperative skin preparation of the foot and ankle: bristles and alcohol are better. J Bone Joint Surg Am 2005;87:986–92.

98. Briggs M. Principles of closed surgical wound care. J Wound Care 1997;6:288–92.

99. Cruse PJ, Foord R. The epidemiology of wound infection. A 10-year prospective study of 62,939 wounds. Surg Clin North Am 1980;60:27–40.

100. Kaul AF, Jewett JF. Agents and techniques for disinfection of the skin. Surg Gynecol Obstet 1981;152:677–85.

101. Alexander JW, Fischer JE, Boyajian M, et al. The influence of hair-removal methods on wound infections. Arch Surg 1983;118:347–52.

102. Balthazar ER, Colt JD, Nichols RL. Preoperative hair removal: a random prospective study of shaving versus clipping. South Med J 1982;75:799–801.

103. Tanner J, Woodings D, Moncaster K. Preoperative hair removal to reduce surgical site infection. Cochrane Database Syst Rev 2006;3:CD004122.

104. Seropian R, Reynolds BM. Wound infections after preoperative depilatory versus razor preparation. Am J Surg 1971;121:251–4.

105. Cheng MT, Chang MC, Wang ST, et al. Efficacy of dilute betadine solution irrigation in the prevention of postoperative infection of spinal surgery. Spine (Phila Pa 1976) 2005;30:1689–93.

106. Roth RM, Gleckman RA, Gantz NM, et al. Antibiotic irrigations. A plea for controlled clinical trials. Pharmacotherapy 1985;5:222–7.

107. Hassinger SM, Harding G, Wongworawat MD. High-pressure pulsatile lavage propagates bacteria into soft tissue. Clin Orthop Relat Res 2005;439:27–31.

108. Kalteis T, Lehn N, Schroder HJ, et al. Contaminant seeding in bone by different irrigation methods: an experimental study. J Orthop Trauma 2005;19:591–6.

109. Bhandari M, Adili A, Lachowski RJ. High pressure pulsatile lavage of contaminated human tibiae: an in vitro study. J Orthop Trauma 1998;12:479–84.

110. Anglen JO. Comparison of soap and antibiotic solutions for irrigation of lower-limb open fracture wounds. A prospective, randomized study. J Bone Joint Surg Am 2005;87:1415–22.

111. Beer KJ, Lombardi AV Jr, Mallory TH, et al. The efficacy of suction drains after routine total joint arthroplasty. J Bone Joint Surg Am 1991;73:584–7.

112. Parker MJ, Roberts CP, Hay D. Closed suction drainage for hip and knee arthroplasty. A meta-analysis. J Bone Joint Surg Am 2004;86:1146–52.

113. Raves JJ, Slifkin M, Diamond DL. A bacteriologic study comparing closed suction and simple conduit drainage. Am J Surg 1984;148:618–20.

114. Sankar B, Ray P, Rai J. Suction drain tip culture in orthopaedic surgery: a prospective study of 214 clean operations. Int Orthop 2004;28:311–4.

115. Drinkwater CJ, Neil MJ. Optimal timing of wound drain removal following total joint arthroplasty. J Arthroplasty 1995;10:185–9.

116. Manian FA, Meyer PL, Setzer J, et al. Surgical site infections associated with methicillin-resistant *Staphylococcus aureus*: do postoperative factors play a role? Clin Infect Dis 2003;36:863–8.

117. Prasarn ML, Zych G, Ostermann PAW. Wound management for severe open fractures: use of antibiotic bead pouches and vacuum-assisted closure. Am J Orthop 2009;38(11):559–63.
118. Morykwas MJ, Simpson J, Punger K, et al. Vacuum-assisted closure: state of basic research and physiologic foundation. Plast Reconstr Surg 2006;117(7 Suppl): 121S–6.
119. White RA, Miki RA, Kazmier P, et al. Vacuum-assisted closure complicated by erosion and hemorrhage of the anterior tibial artery. J Orthop Trauma 2005;19(1): 56–9.
120. Morykwas MJ, Argenta LC, Shelton-Brown EI, et al. Vacuum-assisted closure: a new method for wound control and treatment. Animal studies and basic foundation. Ann Plast Surg 1997;38(6):553–61.
121. Xu L, Chen SZ, Qiao C. Effects of negative pressure on wound blood flow. J Fourth Milit Med Univ 2000;21:967.
122. Agenta LC, Morykwas MJ, Marks MW, et al. Vacuum-assisted closure: state of clinic art. Plast Reconstr Surg 2006;117(7 Suppl):127S–42.
123. DeFranzo AJ, Argenta LC, Marks MW, et al. The use of vacuum-assisted closure therapy for the treatment of lower extremity wounds with exposed bone. Plast Reconstr Surg 2001;108(5):1184–91.
124. Moues CM, Vos MC, van den Bemd GJ, et al. Bacterial load in relation to vacuum-assisted closure wound therapy: a prospective randomized trial. Wound Repair Regen 2004;12(1):11–7.
125. Herscovici D, Sanders RW, Scaduto JM, et al. Vacuum-assisted wound closure therapy (VAC therapy) for the management of patients with high-energy soft tissue injuries. J Orthop Trauma 2003;17(10):683–7.
126. Freeland AE, Senter BS. Septic arthritis and osteomyelitis. Hand Clin 1989;5: 533–52.
127. Abrams RA, Botte MJ. Hand infections: treatment recommendations for specific types. J Am Acad Orthop Surg 1996;4(4):219–30.
128. Boustred AM, Singer M, Hudsen DA, et al. Septic arthritis of the metacarpophalangeal joint and interphalangeal joints of the hand. Ann Plast Surg 1999;42(6):623–8.
129. Sammer DM, Shin AY. Comparison of arthroscopic and open treatment of septic arthritis of the wrist. J Bone Joint Surg Am 2009;91:1387–93.
130. Sinha M, Jain S, Woods DA. Septic arthritis of the small joints of the hand. J Hand Surg Br 2006;31(6):665–72.
131. Chow SP, Pun WK, So YC, et al. Prospective study of 245 open distal fractures of the hand. J Hand Surg Br 1991;16:137
132. Duncan RW, Freeland AF, Jabaley ME, et al. Open hand fractures: an analysis of the recovery of motion and complications. J Hand Surg 1993;18:387.
133. Waldvogel F, Medoff G, Swartz M. Osteomyelitis: a review of clinical features, therapeutic considerations and unusual aspects (second of three parts). N Engl J Med 1970;282:260–6.
134. Termaat MF, Raimakers PGHM, Scholten HJ, et al. The accuracy of diagnostic imaging for the assessment of chronic osteomyelitis: a systematic review and meta-analysis. J Bone Joint Surg Am 2005;87:2464–71.
135. Zalavras CG, Marcus RE, Levin LS, et al. Management of open fractures and subsequent complications. J Bone Joint Surg Am 2007;89(4):884–95.
136. Reilly KE, Linz JC, Stern PJ, et al. Osteomyelitis of the tubular bones of the hand. J Hand Surg Am 1997;22:644–9.
137. Schecter W, Meyer A, Schecter G, et al. Necrotizing fasciitis of the upper extremity. J Hand Surg 1982;7:15–20.

138. Giuliano A, Lewis F, Hadley K. Bacteriology of necrotizing fasciitis. Am J Surg 1977;134:52.
139. Gonzalez MH. Necrotizing fasciitis and gangrene of the upper extremity. Hand Clin 1998;14(4):635–45.
140. Wilkerson R, Paull W, Coville FV. Necrotizing fasciitis: a review of the literature and case report. Clin Orthop 1987;216:187–92.

Index

Note: Page numbers of article titles are in **boldface** type.

A

Abdominal compartment syndrome (ACS), acute bowel injury/acute intestinal distress
  syndrome and, 293–294
    definitions of, 277–278
    intra-abdominal hypertension and, 275, 277–278, 280
    intra-abdominal pressure, during pregnancy, 288–289
      in burn patients, 287–288
      in hematological patients, 288
      in morbidly obese patients, 288
      in pediatric patients, 287
    recognition of, clinical awareness in, 277
      etiology in, 277
    risk factors for, 277, 279
Acute bowel injury, as new concept, 293–294
    defined, 294–295
    vs. intra-abdominal hypertension, 294
Acute intestinal distress syndrome, defined, 294–295
Amino acid(s), arginine
      deficiency of, 184–185
      effects on wound healing, 186–188
      supplementation of, 185–187
    branched-chain, 184
    glutamine, 184
    in wound healing, 183–188
Anesthesia, local, 219, 221
    procedural sedation, 218, 221
    regional, 219
    topical agents, 220
    with nitrous oxide, 232–233
Anger management, wound healing and, 204
Antibiotics, intravenous
      for necrotizing fasciitis, 336
      for osteomyelitis, 335–336
      for septic arthritis, 333–3334
    prophylactic, for bite wounds, 231
      for hand surgery, 328
      for oral injuries, 231
Arginine, as substrate for nitric oxide, 187–188
    deficiency of, 184–185
    effects on wound healing, 186–188
    supplementation of, 185–187

http://dx.doi.org/10.1016/S0899-5885(12)00042-1
0899-5885/12/$ – see front matter © 2012 Elsevier Inc. All rights reserved.
ccnursing.theclinics.com

Printed and bound by CPI Group (UK) Ltd, Croydon, CR0 4YY

03/10/2024

01040445-0018